Vitamins That H

Your Body's Natural Protectors
Vitamin A — defends against infections ...
Vitamin C — battles viruses and bacteria ...
Vitamin B$_6$ — bolsters your immune system ...
Vitamin E — prevents age-related decline ...
Potassium — reduces the risk of stroke ...
Iron — increases your blood ...
There are over 50 vitamins, minerals, and amino acids that can keep you healthy and fit. *Use them!*

How much do you really need? Your body needs only small amounts of vitamins and minerals. But because what the body manufactures is often not enough, these must be obtained from your diet and from supplements. While most books provide limited information, this book shares complete information that you are ever likely to need about vitamins, minerals, and amino acids. The RDA (Recommended Daily Allowance) tables provide expert guidance about the amount of each nutrient you need every day.

The best sources: A balanced diet is the most sensible way of getting a sufficient quantity of these nutrients. The rich and natural sources of all nutrients are listed individually to help you choose the right foods. Some popular myths have been corrected (Spinach is especially rich in iron – *false*. Extra vitamins lengthen your life – *false*) to enable you build a strong immunity system for a healthier, and a more active life.

The Author

H.K. Bakhru enjoys countrywide reputation as a naturopath and popular writer. A member of the Nature Cure Practitioners' Guild, he has made extensive studies on herbs and natural methods of treating diseases. In recognition of his dedication and outstanding contribution in the fields of alternative medicine, he has been honoured with 'Lifetime Achievement Award' and 'Gem of Alternative Medicines' award by the Indian Board of Alternative Medicines, Kolkata.

His well-researched books on nature cure, nutrition, and herbs include *Foods That Heal, Herbs That Heal, Natural Home Remedies for Common Ailments, Health: The Natural Way, A Complete Handbook of Nature Cure, Diet Cure for Common Ailments, A Handbook of Natural Beauty, Nature Cure for Children's Diseases,* and *Natural Health for the Elderly.* In addition, his articles on nature cure, health, nutrition, and herbs appear regularly in newspapers and magazines.

He spends his retired life furthering the cause of nature cure and charitable activities under the auspices of D.H. Bakhru Foundation, a public charitable trust founded and funded by him. He can be contacted at Flat 602, Building 9, Indus Cooperative Housing Society, MHADA HIG Complex, Oshiwara, Andheri (W), Mumbai-400 053. Tel: 639 8779, Fax: 639 8825.

VITAMINS
THAT HEAL
Natural Immunity for
Better Health

H.K. Bakhru

*From The Library Of
Shashi & Beth Ann Miller*

Date _____

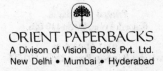

ORIENT PAPERBACKS
A Divison of Vision Books Pvt. Ltd.
New Delhi • Mumbai • Hyderabad

Disclaimer: The information contained in this book is in no way intended to replace professional medical advice and treatment. If you have any doubt or query about the state of your health or you are pregnant, it is advisable to consult and follow your doctor's instructions. The treatments suggested do not normally produce adverse side-effects. However as there are exceptions to the rule, the treatments are to be taken at the reader's sole discretion.

ISBN 81-222-0224-1

1st Published 1998
4th Printing 2002

Vitamins That Heal: Natural Immunity for Better Health

© H.K. Bakhru

Cover design by Vision Studio

Published by
Orient Paperbacks
(A Division of Vision Books Pvt. Ltd.)
Madarsa Road, Kashmere Gate, Delhi-110 006

Printed in India at
Rakesh Press, Delhi-110 028

Cover Printed at
Ravindra Printing Press, Delhi-110 006

CONTENTS

Appendices

An alphabetical list of common ailments which respond to healing properties of vitamins, minerals, and amino acids.

Acidosis—*Lysine*
Acne—*Vitamins A, B_8; Zinc*
Ageing, premature—*Vitamin C, D*
Alcoholism—*Vitamin B_1; Glutamine*
Allergy—*Histidine*
Alopecia—*Vitamins A, B_8, B_9, Inositol; Chlorine, Silicon*
Anaemia—*Vitamins B_2, B_3, B_6, B_8, B_9, B_{12}, C; Calcium, Iodine, Iron, Molybdenum, Zinc; Cystine, Histidine, Lysine*
Angina Pectoris—*See Heart Ailments*
Anorexia—*Vitamins A, B_1, B_8, B_{12}, C*
Anoxia—*Vitamin C*
Appetite, loss of—*Vitamins A, B_1, B_8, B_{12}, C; Lysine*
Arteriosclerosis—*Vitamins B_3, Choline, C; Chromium*
Arthritis—*Vitamins A, B_5, D; Calcium, Copper*
Asthma—*Vitamin A*

Beriberi—*Vitamin B_1*
Biliary Obstruction—*Vitamin K*
Blood Pressure, high—*Vitamins A, B_3, Choline, Inositol, C; Chromium; Gama-Aminobutyric Acid*
Blood Pressure, low—*Vitamin B_5; Iodine; Tyrosine*
Blood Sugar, low—*Vitamin B_5; Potassium; Alanine*
Body Temperature, low—*Tyrosine*
Brain Damage—*Vitamin E; Asparagine, Glutamine*

Cancer—*Vitamin C; Selenium*
Cardiac Ischemia—*See Heart Ailments*
Cardiovascular Disease—*See Heart Ailments*
Cataract—*Vitamin B_2; Selenium; Phenylalanine*

Cerebral Thrombosis—*Vitamin B₃*

Cirrhosis—*See Liver Problems*

Common Cold—*Vitamins A, C*

Congenital Deformities—*Vitamins C, E*

Constipation—*Vitamins B₁, B₅, D; Potassium*

Convulsions—*Vitamins B₆, D*

Cramps—*Vitamin B₅; Calcium*

Cretinism—*Iodine*

Cysts—*Boron*

Dandruff—*Vitamins A, B₈; Selenium*

Dental Problems— *Vitamins A, B₆, C, D; Calcium, Chlorine, Fluorine, Molybdenum; Tryptophan*

Depression— *Vitamins B₁, B₂, B₅, B₆, B₈, B₉, B₁₂; Iron, Magnesium; Glutamine, Tyrosine*

Dermatitis, seborrheic—*See Skin Problems*

Diabetes—*Vitamin B₆; Chromium*

Diarrhoea—*Vitamin B₃*

Digestive Disorders— *Vitamins B₁, B₂, B₃; Chlorine, Copper, Manganese*

Down's Syndrome—*Taurine*

Dysmenorrhoea—*See Menstrual Problems*

Eczema—*Vitamins B₆, B₈, Inositol; Zinc*

Epilepsy— *Chromium, Magnesium; Gama–Aminobutyric Acid, Glutamine*

Excessive Perspiration—*See Skin Problems*

Flatulence—*See Digestive Disorders*

Gastritis—*Inositol*

Genitals, delayed maturation—*Zinc*

Goitre—*Iodine*

Gout—*Vitamin B₉*

Greying, premature—*Vitamins B₅, Inositol; Selenium*

Gum Disorders—*See Dental Problems*

Haematemesis—*Vitamin C*

Haemorrhages—*Vitamin K*

Haemorrhoids—*See Piles*

Hair, loss of—*See Alopecia*

Halitosis—*See Dental Problems*

Headaches—*Vitamin B₃; Lysine*

Hearing Disorders—*Histidine*

Heart Ailments— *Vitamins B_1, B_2, B_3, B_8, Choline, Inositol, E; Calcium, Iodine, Magnesium, Potassium, Selenium; Carnitine, Histidine*

Heat Exhaustion—*Sodium*

Hepatic Coma—*See Liver Problems*

Herpes—*Lysine*

Hyperparathyroidism—*Calcium*

Hypertension—*See Blood Pressure, high*

Hyperthyroidism—*Iodine*

Hypertrophy of the Heart—*See Heart Ailments*

Hypoglycaemia—*See Blood Sugar, low*

Impotence—*Vitamins B_9, E; Manganese, Phosphorus; Arginine*

Infections—*Vitamins B_5, C*

Inflammation, colon—*Vitamin B_6*
　　　　　　　tongue—*Vitamin C*

Influenza—*Vitamin A*

Insomnia—*Vitamins B_1, B_3, B_5, B_6, B_{12}; Calcium; Tryptophan, Valine*

Keshan's Disease—*Selenium*

Kidney Disorders—*Vitamins A, B_6, Choline, C; Calcium, Magnesium; Carnitine, Lysine, Methionine*

Kidney Stones—*See Kidney Disorders*

Liver, fat deposits in the—*See Liver Problems*

Liver Problems—*Choline, Inositol; Selenium, Glutathione, Methionine, Ornithine*

Lung Disease—*See Respiratory Problems*

Malnutrition—*Copper, Chromium; Lysine*

Melanea—*Vitamin C*

Menke's Syndrome—*Copper*

Menopause—*Vitamin E; Calcium, Selenium*

Menstrual Problems—*Vitamin E; Calcium*

Mental Disorders— *Vitamin B_9; Sodium; Glutamine, Phenylalanine, Threonine, Valine*

Mental Retardation—*See Mental Disorders*

Migraine—*Vitamins B_3, B_6*

Miscarriages—*Vitamin E*
Morning Sickness—*See Nausea*
Muscular Disorders—*Vitamins B_6, B_8, E; Sodium,*
Potassium; Carnitine, Valine
Myocardial Infarction—*See Heart Ailments*
Myxoedema—*Iodine*

Nails, imperfect development of—*Sulphur*
Nausea—*Vitamin B_6; Sodium; Lysine*
Nephritis—*See Kidney Disorders*
Nephrosis—*See Kidney Disorders*
Neurasthenia—*See Neurological Problems*
Neuritis—*See Neurological Problems*
Neurological Imbalances—*See Brain Damage*
Neurological Problems—*Vitamins B_1, B_3, B_5, B_6, C;*
Potassium; Tyrosine
Nightblindness—*Vitamin A*
Nose-Bleeding—*Vitamin C*

Obesity—*Cystine*
Oedema—*Vitamins B_1, B_6*
Osteomalacia—*Calcium*
Osteoporosis—*Silicon*

Pellagra—*Vitamin B_3; Tryptophan*
Piles—*Vitamins B_6, C*
Periodontitis—*See Dental Problems*
Pneumonia—*See Respiratory Problems*
Premature Senility—*Vitamin B_6*
Prostrate Disorders—*Zinc*
Protein Energy Malnutrition—*See Malnutrition*
Psychoneurosis—*See Neurological Problems*
Pulmonary Embolism—*See Respiratory Problems*
Pyorrhoea—*See Dental Problems*

Reproductive Disorders—*Vitamins B_9, E*
Restless Feeling in the Legs—*See Neurological Problems*
Respiratory Problems—*Vitamins B_8, E; Copper; Lysine*
Retarded Growth—*Vitamins A, B_5, B_{12}, D; Manganese,*
Phosphorus, Silicon, Zinc
Rheumatic Fever—*Methionine*

Rheumatic Pain—*See Rheumatoid Arthritis*
Rheumatoid Arthritis—*Vitamin B_1; Histidine, Methionine*
Rickets—*Vitamins C, D; Calcium; Lysine*

Schizophrenia—*See Mental Disorders*
Sciatica—*Vitamin B_1; Potassium*
Scurvy—*Vitamin C*
Skin Haemorrhages—*See Skin Problems*
Skin Problems—*Vitamins A, B_2, B_5, B_6, B_8, B_9, C; Magnesium, Potassium, Sulphur, Silicon, Zinc, Cystine, Proline*

Skin—*Zinc*
Sprue—*Vitamin B_9*
Sterility—*Vitamin E; Manganese*
Stress—*See Neurological Problems*
Stroke—*See Brain Damage*

Teeth Formation, defective—*See Dental Problems*
Teeth Loss—*See Dental Problems*
Tetany—*Calcium*
Tooth Decay—*See Dental Problems*
Travel Sickness—*See Nausea*
Tumours—*Boron*

Ulcers, corneal—*Vitamin C*
      duodenal—*Vitamin B_5*
      peptic—*Glutamine*
      skin—*Zinc*
Urinary Problems—*Magnesium*

Varicose Veins—*Vitamin E*

Weight Loss—*Phosphorus, Lysine*
Wounds, healing of—*See Skin Problems*
Wrinkles, premature—*See Skin Problems*

Xerophthalmia—*Vitamin A*

The foods we eat contain vitamins, minerals, and amino acids — the building blocks of proteins, besides other nutrients. These elements contribute greatly towards health and longevity by imparting vigour and vitality to the body, fighting disease and thereby, prolonging life. Sir Robert McCarrison, a well-known nutritionist, aptly remarks, 'The right kind of food is the most important single factor in the promotion of health; and the wrong kind of food is the most important single factor in the promotion of disease.'

The body builds and maintains healthy cells, tissues, glands, and organs with the help of various nutrients that are taken in the diet. The body cannot perform any of its functions, be they metabolic, hormonal, mental, physical, or chemical, without them.

Food is also of utmost importance in the cure of disease. The primary cause of disease is a weakened organism or lowered resistance in the body, arising from the adoption of faulty food habits. There is an elaborate healing mechanism within the body but it can perform its function only if it is abundantly supplied with all the essential nutritional factors. It is believed that about 45 chemical components and elements are needed by human cells. Each of these 45 substances — carbohydrates, proteins, fats, minerals, and vitamins — must be present in the diet.

Vitamins and minerals, though required in small quantities, govern many vital functions connected with metabolism, reproduction, the immune mechanism, and intelligence. Certain vitamins also possess antioxidant properties which reduce oxidation and counter the damaging effects of free radicals in the body and prevent oxidation process. These vitamins are A,E,C, and B-carotene. By virtue of their properties, they can delay the ageing process. They also prevent degeneration in blood vessels, heart joints, and the lenses of the eyes.

Protein is one of the most important nutrients needed by the body. It is the very basis of life, and the only food substance that can repair and rebuild cells, thus restoring health and prolonging life. Amino acids, the building-blocks of protein, therefore play a vital role in the maintenance of good health.

Research has shown that almost all varieties of disease can be produced by an inadequate supply of vitamins, minerals, amino acids, and other nutrients. These nutritional deficiencies occur on account of several factors. The most important of these factors is the intense processing and refining of foods like cereals and sugar. This results in a colossal loss of vitamins, minerals, and other nutrients and is responsible, to a large extent, for the vast array of present-day diseases.

For instance, wheat is an excellent health-building food, with its essential coating of bran, vitamins, and minerals. But refining it in mills leads to a loss of the essential wheat germ, vitamins, and minerals, resulting in constipation and other digestive disturbances and nutritional disorders.

Similarly, the heat and chemical processes employed in the refining of sugar kill the vitamins and separate the minerals, protein and other substances from the sap, leaving nothing but pure sugar crystals which are difficult to digest. High intake of refined white sugar can rob the body of the vitamins supplied to it through other foods. It can also cause gastric catarrh, hyperacidity, and tooth decay.

Another factor which leads to deficiencies of vitamins and minerals is the time lag between the harvesting and consumption of vegetables and fruits. Further loss of these nutrients occurs due to the storage, paring, and grating of vegetables, soaking them in water, and from the heat of cooking.

This book describes at some length the important functions which various vitamins, minerals, and amino acids perform in the body and the serious consequences of their deficiencies. It also provides information about their valuable food sources, their recommended intake, and their therapeutic uses in treating specific diseases. A diet which contains liberal quantities of seeds, nuts and grains, vegetables, and fruits provides adequate amounts of all the essential nutrients. I earnestly hope that this knowledge will greatly benefit readers. By putting it into practice, they can maintain good health, ward off disease, and prolong their life span.

If you eat a varied and well-balanced diet, you are probably getting adequate amounts of nutrients, including the vitamins and minerals you need for good health. However, sometimes vitamin and mineral supplements are necessary. For example, babies need extra vitamin D in infancy. Folic acid supplements are given to women during pregnancy. Supplementary vitamins and minerals are useful after an illness, surgery or while recuperating from any incident which interferes, over time, with eating normal, balanced meals.

Recommended Daily Allowance(RDA): The average daily requirements of vitamins, minerals, and amino acids given in the book are based on guidelines developed by the National Institute of Nutrition, Indian Council of Medical Research, and other organisations involved in nutrition programmes. The RDA is the quantity we require unless a supplement has been prescribed, in which case the doctor's instructions must be followed; otherwise the commonsense guidelines given in the book are sufficient.

The categorisation of age groups used in the RDAs is:

Infants	upto 12 months
Children	1-to-14 years
Adults	14 years of age and above

The RDAs and amounts of nutrients present in foods are given in micrograms(mcg), milligrams(mg), or grams(g).

1,000 micrograms	=	1 milligram
1,000 milligrams	=	1 gram

Remember your objective is a *balanced* and *adequate* intake of all nutrients, including vitamins, minerals, and amino acids, to maintain and sustain good health.

PART I
Vitamins for Healthy Living

*Life is not living,
but living in health.*
—*Martial*

The science of nutrition changed drastically in 1906 with the research findings of British biochemist F. G. Hopkins. After six years of extensive research, he came to the conclusion that, apart from organic and inorganic food components, there were certain other chemical substances in organic form which were present in natural foods and were essential for normal metabolic functions in human beings and other animals. These were indispensable for the health and growth of body cells and protection against infective and degenerative diseases.

Six years later, these mysterious substances were given a name. A Polish chemist, Casimir Funk, while working at the Lister Institute in London, isolated a chemical compound, an amine, which he used to cure beriberi disease in experiments with pigeons. Funk suggested that a whole family of amine compounds played a vital role in nutrition and the lack of any of them could lead to fatal illness. Funk proposed that the whole family be called Vitamines, from *vita*, the Latin word for 'life', plus *amine*. Later research showed that not all such substances were amines, and to prevent confusion, the final 'e' was dropped to create the modern word Vitamin.

E. V. McCollum, at the University of Wisconsin, USA, began further investigation of Hopkins' discovery of the growth-promoting factors in milk. He separated milk into its fat and water portions to find out which portion of the milk contained the growth-promoting factor. He called the fat portion, Fat-soluble A, and the water portion, Water-soluble B. Both had vitamin action, and Water-soluble B was found to have the same action as thiamine. Thus, in 1913, it was presumed that there were only two vitamins. However it soon became apparent that there were far more than just two vitamins. Today, more than two dozen of them are recognised.

When taken in correct amounts and regularly, vitamins are responsible for good health and vitality, energy, growth, and longevity. They are found in small concentrations in foods. With a few exceptions, they cannot be manufactured or synthesised by organisms and their absence or improper absorption results in specific deficiency diseases.

Each of the essential vitamins has a specific function in the body. However, individually, none of them can work efficiently. They are effective only when they work with one another and in combination with carbohydrates, fats, and proteins that are provided by a nutritious diet. They fight infections, maintain the body's natural immune system and help in tissue and bone formation.

The use of vitamins was developed further on account of the research done after the Second World War. People came to know of their wonderful life-sustaining effect on the human body during health and disease, and started taking them for every problem. This excessive consumption of vitamins attracted the attention of chemists who began to analyse their structure. After several years of research, they finally succeeded. Today, all vitamins in use are synthetic: they can be easily manufactured in huge amounts and dispensed in various forms like tablets, capsules, syrups, and injections under a large variety of names and brands.

Vitamins differ from each other in physiological function, in chemical structure, and in distribution in food. They are broadly divided into two categories: fat-soluble and water-soluble. Vitamins A, D, E, and K are all soluble in fat and fat solvents and are known as fat-soluble. They are not easily lost by ordinary cooking methods and they can be stored in the body to some extent, mostly in the liver. Vitamin B complex and C are water-soluble. They dissolve easily in cooking water. A portion of these vitamins may actually be destroyed by heating. They cannot be stored in the body and hence, have to be taken daily in foods. Any extra quantity taken on any one day is eliminated as waste.

Used therapeutically, vitamins can be of immense help in treating disease and speeding recovery. They can be used in two ways: correcting deficiencies and treating diseases. Latest research indicates that many vitamins taken in large doses, far above the actual nutritional needs, can heal a wide range of common complaints and illnesses. Vitamin therapy has a distinct advantage over drug therapy: while drugs are always toxic and have many undesirable side-effects, vitamins, as a rule, are non-toxic and safe.

The various functions of common vitamins, their deficiency symptoms, natural sources, daily requirements, and their therapeutic uses are discussed in the following chapters.

For Better Eyesight

The first nutritional deficiency disease to be clearly recognised was, probably, nightblindness. The ancient Egyptians, as mentioned in the *Papyrus Ebers* and later in the *London Medical Papyrus*, recommended that juice extracted

Recommended Daily Allowance		
Men	600	mcg
Women	600	mcg
Lact. Wo.*	950	mcg
Children	600	mcg
Infants	350	mcg

from cooked liver should be applied to the eye to cure nightblindness. Though these writings date to 1,500 B.C., the observations were probably of much earlier origin. The ancient Greeks, who followed Egyptian medical practices, recommended both the ingestion of cooked liver and its external application as a cure for nightblindness.

Although interesting references to vitamin A-deficiency diseases and their cure can be found throughout history, it was only in 1913 that this vitamin was recognised as the first fat-soluble vitamin and an essential nutrient for growth and survival. In that year, two groups of researchers, E. V. McCollum and Marguerite Davis at the University of Wisconsin, and T. B. Osborne and L. B. Mendel at Yale, demonstrated independently that a fat-soluble factor present in butter was essential for the growth of rats on a synthetic diet. In 1930, T. Moore made the important discovery that when carotene, a pigment present in carrots and other vegetables and fruits, was fed to vitamin A-deficient

---

* Lact. Wo. — Lactating Women.

rats, vitamin A was found in the liver. Carotene is a yellow pigment found in vegetable foods. It is converted into vitamin A in the body.

Vitamin A or retinol is found in foods of animal origin, while carotene is provided by foods of both plant and animal origin. Vitamin A can either be ingested or synthesised within the body from plant carotene. Those whose intake of vitamin A is only in the form of carotene should take a daily recommended amount as follows: Men: 2,400 mcg; Women: 2,400 mcg; Lactation: 3,800 mcg; Children: 1,600-2,400 mcg; Infants: 1,200 mcg. As a concentrated solution, retinol is light yellow in colour. It solidifies when cooled and has a mild pleasant odour. It is insoluble in water or glycerol but soluble in most organic solvents. It is sensitive to oxidation by air in the presence of light.

Approximately 80 per cent of vitamin A is absorbed in the human system. It is passed along with fat through the lymphatic system into the bloodstream. The absorption of vitamin A increases if it is taken with fats. Absorption is more rapid in men than in women. The absorption of this vitamin is poor in cases of diarrhoea, jaundice, and abdominal disorders. Vitamin A is stored in the liver. A healthy person can store about 97.2 mcg of vitamin A per g of liver. Thus an average liver weighing 1,500 g can store 1,50,000 mcg of vitamin A.

Approximately 20 per cent of vitamin A which is not absorbed is excreted within one or two days into the faeces. Of the 80 per cent absorbed, about 20 to 50 per cent either combines with or burns down into products that are excreted within about one week in the faeces or urine. The remainder 30 to 60 per cent of the absorbed vitamin A is stored.

Functions in the Body

The best-defined function of vitamin A is its role in vision. It provides the required stimulation for vision in the retina. In addition, vitamin A is required for growth, reproduction, and the maintenance of life. It builds up resistance to respiratory and other infections, and keeps the mucous linings and membranes of the body, especially those of the eyes, lungs, stomach, and intestines, in a healthy condition. It prevents eye diseases, aids in the secretion of gastric juices, and the digestion of protein. It also plays a vital role in preventing and clearing up infections of the skin, and in promoting healthy hair, teeth, and gums. Vitamin A increases the permeability of blood capillaries, thereby contributing better tissue oxygenation. It also helps prevent premature ageing and senility, increases life expectancy, and extends youthfulness.

Sources

Foods rich in vitamin A(retinol) include those of animal origin such as sheep liver, egg yolk, wholemilk, butter, and *ghee*. Vegetables such as colocasia, turnip greens, drumsticks, beet, carrots, and spinach contain a lot of carotene. Fruits like mangoes, apricots, gooseberries, raspberries, and oranges are also rich in carotene.

Deficiency Symptoms

Prolonged deficiency of vitamin A may result in inflammation of the eyes, poor vision, and nightblindness. There is an increased susceptibility to infections, especially of the respiratory tract, in the form of frequent and prolonged common colds. Vitamin A deficiency may lead to lack of appetite and vigour, defective teeth and gums, skin disorders such as pimples, acne, boils, and premature wrinkles. When vitamin A is present in insufficient amounts, the mucous membranes of the

Rich Sources of Vitamin A(Carotene and Retinol)*

Cereals & Pulses**	mcg
Red gram, tender	469
Soya beans	426
Lentil	270
Bengal gram, whole	189
Bajra	132
Split red gram	132
Split Bengal gram	129
Split Kesari	120

Vegetables & Nuts**	
Colocasia leaves, black variety	12,000
Colocasia leaves, green variety	10,278
Turnip greens	9,396
Drumstick leaves	6,780
Beet greens	5,862
Betel leaves	5,760
Carrot leaves	5,700
Spinach	5,580
Amaranth, tender gangeticus	5,520
Radish leaves	5,295
Celery leaves	3,990
Fenugreek leaves	2,340
Parsley	1,920
Carrots	1,890
Bathua leaves	1,740
Lettuce	990
Onion stalks	595
Pistachio nuts	144

Fruits**	mcg
Mangoes, ripe	2,743
Persimmon	2,268
Apricots, fresh	2,160
Passion fruit juice	1,968
Cape gooseberries	1,428
Raspberries	1,248
Oranges	1,104
Papayas, ripe	666
Loquats	559
Tomatoes, ripe	351
Jack fruit	175
Melons, musk	169
Plums	166
Figs	162

Meat, Poultry, Milk & Milk Products***	
Liver, sheep	6,690
Eggs	420
Wholemilk powder, cow's milk	420
Khoa, wholemilk, cow's	149
Cottage cheese, cow's milk	110

Fats & Edible Oils***	
Butter	960
Hydrogenated oil, fortified	750
Ghee, cow	600
Ghee, buffalo	270

* Values per 100 g edible portions.
** These values represent mcg of Carotene.
*** These values represent mcg of vitamin A(Retinol).

nose, throat, and mouth, the bronchial tubes, lungs, intestinal tract, kidneys, and vagina are greatly affected. Eventually the mucous membranes of the entire body lose their ability to secrete the normal quantities of mucus needed to protect them from irritation, and the body degenerates rapidly. Other deficiency symptoms include retarded growth in children, dry and dull hair, dandruff, excessive hair loss, ridged nails, and a poor sense of taste and smell.

Healing and Therapeutic Properties

When taken in large therapeutic doses of 7,500 mcg to 15,000 mcg a day, for purposes of treating deficiency conditions, vitamin A is beneficial in the treatment of common colds, sinus problems, influenza and other infectious diseases. Vitamin A is valuable in curing nightblindness and other eye diseases, as well as asthma, arthritis, high blood pressure, and kidney disorders.

Eye Problems. Nightblindness and the milder conjuctival changes respond well to 9,000 mcg of vitamin A daily for a week. Corneal damage constitutes a therapeutic emergency, and the usual treatment is 6,000 mcg per kg of body weight, per day, for 5 days.

Larger doses of vitamin A have been used for reducing the incidence of vitamin A deficiency in small children. In cases of xerophthalmia, a type of dry conjuctivitis due to lack of vitamin A in very young children, 60,000 mcg of retinol can be administered orally in a single dose with beneficial results. The dose can be repeated every six months without any ill effects.

Acne. Vitamin A therapy has been found beneficial in the treatment of acne. A generous intake of this vitamin is needed for this purpose. Adelle Davis, the world-famous nutritionist, says that she has seen many stubborn cases of acne clear up when nutrition has included an adequate amount of vitamin A.

Other Skin Disorders. It is believed that intake of vitamin A in large doses helps relieve warts and other growths in the skin such as boils, rashes, and carbuncles. Depending upon the condition of the skin, the intake may vary from 7,500—15,000 mcg per day for one month. Vitamin A therapy is considered especially effective for corns.

Precautions. More than 30,000 mcg of vitamin A taken daily can produce toxic effects in adults if continued for many months. In infants, toxic effects can be produced by the intake of more than 5,550 mcg per day. Toxicity symptoms include hair loss, nausea, vomiting, diarrhoea, scaly skin, blurred vision, rashes, pain in the bones, irregular menstruation, fatigue, headache, and liver enlargement. Acute toxicity from a single massive dose manifests itself as abdominal pain, nausea, vomiting, headache, dizziness, and sluggishness. Chronic toxicity may occur following ingestion of 12,000 mcg or more daily for prolonged periods. It is characterised by joint pains — more especially of the feet, hair loss, dryness and fissures of the lips, loss of appetite, low-grade fever, and weight loss.

For Calm Nerves

Vitamin B_1 or thiamine, as it is more commonly referred to now, is one of the most important members of the B group of vitamins. Also known as aneurin, vitamin B_1 is anti-beriberi and anti-neuritic. It is water-soluble.

Recommended Daily Allowance	
Men	1.3 mg
Women	1.0 mg
Children	1.1 mg
Infants	50 mcg*

Vitamin B_1 was discovered by Eijkman, a Dutch physician, in 1897, while working in a military hospital in Java. He noticed that the poultry at the prison hospital showed symptoms similar to those of his patients suffering from beriberi, a debilitating condition. This malady developed in the chickens when they were fed on table scraps of polished rice. Recovery followed when they were fed on brown rice. Eijkman showed that there was something existing in very small amounts in the germ and pericarp(layer surrounding the grain) of rice that protected fowl from a disease resembling beriberi: he admitted that it was an unknown nutrient. Thirty years later, Jansen and Donath, working in the same laboratory, succeeded in isolating this factor in crystalline form: it came to be known as thiamine. In 1934, Williams and his co-workers made improvements in the methods of isolation of thiamine.

Vitamin B_1 in the form of thiamine hydrochloride, is a white crystalline powder with a yeast-like odour and a saltish taste. It is readily soluble in water and slightly

* Value per kg of body weight.

soluble in alcohol. In dry form, this vitamin is very stable and not sensitive to atmospheric oxidation or deterioration. However, in a soluble form, it is destroyed soon.

Heat applied in cooking destroys this vitamin. The loss is significant when vegetables are cooked in excessive water which is thrown away afterwards. The addition of sodium carbonate(cooking soda) in some vegetables further increases the destruction of this vitamin. Thiamine is well retained in cereals, since they are generally cooked slowly and at moderate temperatures; the cooking water is also retained. Baked products lose about 15 per cent of their original thiamine. Generally the losses in cooking meat are greater than in cooking other foods, ranging from 25 to 50 per cent of the raw value. Other destroyers of thiamine are caffeine, alcohol, food-processing methods, and sulphur drugs.

Thiamine is absorbed from the small intestine. The capacity of the human intestine to absorb this vitamin is limited to about 5 mg per day. Thiamine undergoes a change in the intestinal mucosa. Approximately 25 to 30 mg are stored in this changed form in the body. Large amounts of thiamine are present in the skeletal muscles, heart, liver, kidneys, and brain. This vitamin cannot, however, be stored to any large extent in the human body. So an adequate daily intake is necessary. Any excess supply of thiamine is excreted in the urine.

Functions in the Body

Thiamine promotes growth, protects the heart muscle, and stimulates brain action. It plays an important role in the normal functioning of the entire nervous system. It aids digestion, especially of carbohydrates. It has a mild diuretic effect: that is, it increases urine formation.

This vitamin improves peristalsis and helps to prevent constipation. It also helps to maintain the normal red blood count, improves circulation, and promotes a healthy skin. It protects against the damaging effect of lead poisoning, and prevents oedema or fluid retention in connection with heart ailments. It also reduces fatigue, increases stamina, and prevents premature ageing and senility by increasing mental alertness. Like other vitamins of the B complex group, it is more potent when combined with other B vitamins rather than when used separately.

Sources

Wholegrain cereals, especially wheat, rice, and oats, are generally considered to be the best sources of thiamine. Thiamine is usually found in the germ and outer layers. However, when these grains are highly refined, for example, as white flour and polished rice, the amount of thiamine is considerably reduced. Legumes such as soya beans and Bengal gram are good sources of thiamine. Other good sources of this vitamin are vegetables such as dry lotus stems, capsicum, turnip greens, and beet greens; fruits such as apricots and pineapples; nuts such as groundnuts, pistachio nuts, and mustard seeds; and animal foods like pork, sheep liver, and mutton.

Deficiency Symptoms

A lack of sufficient thiamine in the diet can cause loss of appetite, poor digestion, chronic constipation, loss of weight, mental depression, nervous exhaustion, and insomnia. It can lead to muscular weakness, leg cramps, slow heartbeat, irritability, defective hydrochloric acid production in the stomach and consequent digestive disorders. In case of insufficient supply of thiamine in the body, the heart muscles become lazy and fatigued,

Rich Sources of Vitamin B₁ (Thiamine)*

Cereals	mcg	Nuts & Oilseeds	mcg
Rice bran	2,700	Groundnuts	900
Wheat germ	1,400	Pistachio nuts	670
Wheat flour, whole	490	Mustard seeds	650
Barley	470	Cashew nuts	630
Maize, dry	420	Walnuts	450
Finger millet	420	Chilgozas	320
Bajra	330	Almonds	240
Rice, parboiled, hand-pounded	270	**Fruits**	
		Apricots, dried	220
Pulses & Legumes		Pineapples	200
Soya beans	730	Bael fruit	130
Split Bengal gram	480	Melons, musk	110
Split green gram	470		
Peas, roasted	470	**Meat & Poultry**	
Lentil	450	Pork	540
Moth beans	450	Liver, sheep	360
Split red gram	450	Mutton	180
Split black gram	420	Beef, muscle, lean	150
Red gram, tender	320	Eggs	100
Vegetables		**Milk & Milk Products**	
Lotus stems, dry	820	Skimmed milk powder, cow's milk	450
Capsicums	550		
Turnip greens	310	Wholemilk powder, cow's milk	310
Beet greens	260		
Colocasia leaves, green variety	220	*Khoa*, wholemilk, cow's	230
Radish leaves	180		
Potatoes	100		

* Values per 100 g edible portions.

---

and the auricles or the upper chambers of the heart lose their strength and gradually enlarge. This may lead to a condition known as hypertrophy of the heart. Prolonged gross deficiency can cause beriberi, neuritis, and oedema. Lack of vitamin B₁ can slow down circulation to the scalp to the extent that hair may fall and new hair may grow very slowly. Deficiency of thiamine can be induced by excessive use of alcohol, dietary sugar, and processed and refined foods.

Healing and Therapeutic Properties

Taken in large therapeutic doses of upto 50,000 mcg a day, thiamine is beneficial in the treatment of constipation and other digestive disorders, neuritis and other nervous troubles, as well as mental depression. It is life saving in the treatment of cardiovascular disease related to beriberi and infantile beriberi. Thiamine is also used with beneficial results in the treatment of alcoholism, insomnia, and stress.

Beriberi. Prompt administration of thiamine is indicated when beriberi is diagnosed or suspected. Fifty thousand micrograms per day should be given intramuscularly for several days. Thereafter, 2,500 to 5,000 mcg per day can be administered by mouth. Larger amounts are usually not absorbed. Patients should also receive other water-soluble vitamins in therapeutic quantities.

A simple way to treat infantile beriberi is via the mother's milk. The mother should receive 10,000 mcg of thiamine twice daily; in severe cases this should be given by injection. In addition, the infant should be given thiamine in doses of upto 10,000 to 20,000 mcg intramuscularly, once a day, for three days. This should be followed by 5,000 to 10,000 mcg orally, twice a day. When symptoms of heart failure are present, or there are convulsions or coma, the initial dose may be increased from 25,000 to 50,000 mcg given intravenously and very slowly. Thereafter treatment should be by intramuscular injection, followed by oral therapy.

Nervous Disorders. Vitamin B_1 is indispensable for the metabolism of carbohydrates, and the cells of the nervous system are entirely dependent on carbohydrates for their energy requirement. The primary role of vitamin B_1 is to ensure energy for nerve cells and to protect them from harm. This vitamin is used therapeutically in neurological disorders with muscular weakness and cramps. It is particularly useful in all painful conditions like neuritis and polyneuritis, rheumatic neuralgias, sciatica, and rheumatic pain.

Heart Disease. Studies indicate that vitamin B_1 deficiency may complicate existing heart disease. Therapeutic doses of vitamin B_1 have been found especially beneficial in beriberi-related heart disease which is caused by gross malnutrition and is commonly prevalent in chronic alcoholics. Improvement can be affected in such cases by bedrest, a high-carbohydrate-cum-high-protein diet, and 200 mg or 200,000 mcg of vitamin B_1 given thrice daily by injection. After some improvement is seen, further progress can be made by continuing the same diet and an oral intake of 50 mg or 50,000 mcg of thiamine thrice daily.

Gastro-Intestinal Disorders. In various gastro-intestinal disorders, 50,000 mcg of vitamin B_1 given three times a day immediately after meals, with a suitable digestive enzyme preparation, is found to be very effective. It is particularly useful for carbohydrate and protein indigestion, loss of appetite, flatulence, constipation, and abdominal distension.

Precautions. There is no known toxic effect of thiamine. Any excess is excreted in the urine and not stored in any degree in the tissues or organs. However rare symptoms of overdose include tremors, herpes, oedema, nervousness, rapid heartbeat, and allergies. In rare cases excessive supply of this vitamin may also adversely affect thyroid and insulin production.

The 'Beauty' Vitamin

Vitamin B_2 or riboflavin is the second member of the B complex group. The word riboflavin is derived from two sources: *ribose*, referring to ribose sugar found in several vitamins and enzymes, and *flavin* meaning yellow. Since that part of

Recommended Daily Allowance	
Men	1.5 mg
Women	1.2 mg
Children	1.3 mg
Infants	60 mcg*

the B complex vitamins which remained intact even after heating, contained a molecule similar to that of ribose sugar and was yellow in colour, it came to be known as riboflavin.

This vitamin was recognised in the 1920s when it became evident that some growth-promoting properties of vitamin B were retained after heat had destroyed the anti-beriberi properties. This B factor was finally isolated from milk by Kuhn and his colleagues in 1933, when they succeeded in extracting one gram of crystalline riboflavin from 5,400 litres of whey.

Riboflavin is a crystalline compound with a beautiful yellow-orange hue. It is soluble in water. Though readily decomposed by heat in an alkaline solution, it is not destroyed by boiling in an acid solution. This vitamin is very sensitive to both visible and ultraviolet light. Considerable loss may occur if foods are exposed to light. Thus sun-drying of foods destroys most of their riboflavin content. Ordinary cooking does not affect riboflavin, but cooking in a large quantity of

* Value per kg of body weight.

water causes some of this vitamin to be drained out from the food. Sulpha drugs and alcohol can destroy vitamin B_2.

Riboflavin is absorbed into the bloodstream through the walls of the small intestine. It is carried to the tissues of the body and incorporated into the cell enzymes. The liver is the major site of storage and it contains about one-third of the total riboflavin in the body. The liver, kidneys, and heart have the richest concentrations of this vitamin. However the body does not store large quantities of it. Riboflavin is excreted primarily in the urine. Bile and sweat are other minor routes of excretion.

Functions in the Body

Riboflavin is essential for growth and general health. It functions as a part of a group of enzymes which are involved in the metabolism of carbohydrates, fats, and proteins. It is involved in a number of chemical reactions in the body and is therefore essential for normal tissue maintenance.

Riboflavin aids digestion and helps in the functioning of the nervous system. It prevents constipation, promotes a healthy skin, nails, and hair, and strengthens the mucous lining of the mouth, lips, and tongue. Riboflavin also plays an important role in the health of the eyes and alleviates eye strain. This vitamin is particularly helpful in counteracting the tendency towards glaucoma. An ample supply of vitamin B_2 provides vigour and helps to preserve the appearance and feeling of youth.

Sources

Riboflavin, though widely distributed in vegetable and animal foods, is present only in small amounts in most of them. Foods rich in riboflavin are green vegetables such as lotus stems, turnip greens, beets, radish leaves, colocasia and carrot leaves; fruits such as papaya, raisins, custard apples and apricots; foods of animal origin such as sheep liver and eggs, skimmed and wholemilk powder of cow's milk and *khoa*. Other well-known sources of this vitamin are almonds, walnuts, chilgozas, pistachio nuts, and mustard seeds. An average person may not be able to get an optimum amount of riboflavin unless he consumes a generous amount of milk. Milling of rice and wheat results in considerable loss of riboflavin since most of the vitamin is present in the germ and bran, which are removed during this process.

Deficiency Symptoms

A deficiency of riboflavin may result in bloodshot eyes, abnormal sensitivity to light, itching and burning of the eyes, inflammation in the mouth, a sore and burning tongue, and cracks on the lips and in the corners of the mouth. It may also result in dull or oily hair, an oily skin, premature wrinkles on the face and arms, and split nails. Riboflavin deficiency also leads to the malfunctioning of the adrenal glands. It can be a contributing cause to such disorders as anaemia, vaginal itching, and cataract.

Healing and Therapeutic Properties

The intake of riboflavin in larger quantities from 25 to 50 mg or 25,000 to 50,000 mcg is beneficial in the treatment of nutritional deficiencies, cataract and other eye ailments, digestive disturbances, nervous depression, and general debility.

Cataract. Riboflavin holds out hope for the victims of a type of cataract known as Nutritional Cataract. This was discovered in a study at the University of Georgia Medical School: riboflavin was found to be extremely beneficial in preventing cataract or checking its further

Rich Sources of Vitamin B₂ (Riboflavin)*

Cereals	mcg	Nuts & Oilseeds	mcg
Wheat germ	540	Almonds	570
Rice bran	480	Walnuts	400
Bajra	250	Chilgozas	300
Barley	200	Pistachio nuts	280
Finger millet	190	Mustard seeds	260
Wheat flour, whole	170	Cashew nuts	190
Rice, parboiled, hand-pounded	120	Groundnuts	130
Pulses & Legumes		**Fruits**	
Soya beans	390	Papayas, ripe	250
Red gram, tender	330	Raisins	190
Split green gram	210	Custard apples	170
Peas, roasted	210	Currants, black	140
Split black gram	200	Apricots, fresh	130
Lentil	200	Jack fruit	130
Split red gram	190	Pineapples	120
Split Bengal gram	180	**Fish, Sea Foods, Meat & Poultry**	
Vegetables		Liver, sheep	1,700
Lotus stems, dry	1,210	Eggs	400
Turnip greens	570	Pomfret, white	150
Beet greens	560	Mutton	140
Radish leaves	470	Prawn	100
Colocasia leaves, black variety	450	**Milk & Milk Products**	
Carrot leaves	370	Skimmed milk powder, cow's milk	1,640
Fenugreek leaves	310	Wholemilk powder, cow's milk	1,360
Spinach	260	*Khoa*, wholemilk, cow's	410
Brussels sprouts	160	Milk, cow's	190
Bathua leaves	140	Curd, cow's milk	160
Lettuce	130	Milk, buffalo's	100
Brinjals	110		
Cauliflower	100		

* Values per 100 g edible portions.

growth. Anyone whose eye muscles are weak or who has eye trouble of any sort, including cataract, or who fears the possibility of cataract, should include large amounts of riboflavin in the diet in consultation with his physician. While vitamin A is concerned with the vision in the eye, riboflavin strengthens the muscles and nerves of the eye.

Skin Problems. Skin complaints such as oiliness, whiteheads, blackheads, scaling, cracks, and sores can often be cleared by taking riboflavin in therapeutic doses. Even a mild lack of this vitamin over a long time causes brown pigmentation of the skin. If generous amounts of vitamin B_2, to the extent of 15 mg or 15,000 mcg are taken daily over a period of six months, these ugly spots usually disappear.

Precautions. Riboflavin has a low level of toxicity and no case of toxicity from riboflavin has been reported in humans. This is probably because the transport system necessary for the absorption of riboflavin across the gastro-intestinal mucosa becomes saturated, limiting the amount of the vitamin that can be absorbed. Possible symptoms of minor excess include itching, numbness, a sensation of burning, or pricking.

Relieves Skin Eruptions

Vitamin B_3 or niacin is an important vitamin of the B group. From 1867 it was known as nicotinic acid to organic chemists. As early as 1913, Funk isolated it from yeast. However it attracted attention only in 1937, when C. A.

Recommended Daily Allowance	
Men	17 mg
Women	13 mg
Children	15 mg
Infants	650 mcg*

Elvehjem and his colleagues isolated it from the liver. Later, T. W. Spies and others demonstrated that most of the classic symptoms of pellagra, diarrhoea, and mental derangement were relieved with the administration of niacin.

Although nicotinic acid is chemically related to nicotine found in tobacco, it has none of its physiological properties. It is, therefore, commonly called niacin to avoid confusion. Niacin is an odourless, white, crystalline substance, readily soluble in water. It is resistant to heat, oxidation, and alkalies. It is, in fact, one of the most stable vitamins.

Cooking causes little actual destruction of niacin, but a considerable amount may be lost in the cooking water and drippings from cooked meat if these are discarded. In a mixed diet, 15 to 25 per cent of niacin of the cooked foodstuff may be lost in this way. Sulphur drugs, alcohol, food-processing techniques, and sleeping pills tend to destroy this vitamin.

Niacin is absorbed from both the stomach and

* Value per kg of body weight.

intestines and stored in all the tissues. It is excreted in the urine, mostly as its salts, and to a smaller extent, as free niacin.

Functions in the Body

Niacin is important for proper blood circulation and the healthy functioning of the nervous system. It maintains the normal functions of the gastro–intestinal tract and is essential for the proper metabolism of proteins and carbohydrates. It helps to maintain a healthy skin. Niacin dilates the blood vessels and increases the flow of blood to the peripheral capillary system. This vitamin is also essential for synthesis of the sex hormones, namely, oestrogen, progesterone, and testosterone, as well as cortisone, thyroxin, and insulin.

Sources

In general, meat and fish are better sources of niacin than plant products. Foods of animal origin rich in this vitamin are sheep liver, lean meats, prawns, pork, and cow's milk. Vegetarian sources rich in this vitamin are rice bran, rice, wheat, groundnuts, sunflower seeds, almonds, and chilgozas; and green vegetables like turnip and beet greens, and the leaves of carrots, colocasia, and celery. Yeast and bran are good natural sources of this vitamin but the removal of the bran in the milling of wheat reduces the niacin content of white-wheat flour to a low level.

Deficiency Symptoms

A mild deficiency of niacin may result in a coated tongue, sores in the mouth, irritability, nervousness, skin lesions, diarrhoea, forgetfulness, insomnia, chronic headaches, digestive disorders, and anaemia. Severe prolonged deficiency may cause neurasthenia (weakness of the nerves), mental disturbances, depression, mental dullness, and disorientation.

Rich Sources of Vitamin B_3 (Niacin)*

Cereals	*mcg*
Rice bran	29,800
Barley	5,400
Wheat flour, whole	4,300
Rice, puffed	4,100
Rice, flakes	4,000
Rice, parboiled, hand-pounded	4,000
Rice, parboiled, milled	3,800
Jowar	3,100
Wheat germ	2,900
Bajra	2,300
Maize, dry	1,800
Finger millet	1,100
Pulses & Legumes	
Peas, roasted	3,500
Soya beans	3,200
Red gram, tender	3,000
Bengal gram, whole	2,900
Split kesari	2,900
Split red gram	2,900
Lentil	2,600
Split Bengal gram	2,400
Split green gram	2,400
Split black gram	2,000
Moth beans	1,500
Vegetables	
Turnip greens	5,400
Beet greens	3,300
Carrot leaves	2,100
Colocasia leaves, black variety	1,900
Lotus stems, dry	1,900
Celery leaves	1,200
Potatoes	1,200

Nuts & Oilseeds	*mcg*
Groundnuts, roasted	22,100
Sunflower seeds	4,500
Almonds	4,400
Mustard seeds	4,000
Chilgozas	3,600
Coconut, dry	3,000
Pistachio nuts	2,300
Cashew nuts	1,200
Walnuts	1,000
Fruits	
Apricots, dried	2,300
Passion fruit	1,600
Custard apples	1,300
Bael fruit	1,100
Dates, dried	900
Mangoes, ripe	900
Fish, Sea Food & Meat	
Liver, sheep	17,600
Mutton	6,800
Beef, lean	6,400
Prawns	4,800
Indian shard	2,800
Pork	2,800
Pomfret, white	2,600
Sardines	2,600
Milk & Milk Products	
Skimmed milk powder, cow's milk	1,000
Wholemilk powder, cow's milk	800

* Values per 100 g edible portions.

Healing and Therapeutic Properties

Large doses of upto 100 mg or 100,000 mcg of niacin with each meal, preferably taken together with other B group vitamins, provide tremendous relief in cases of pellagra, migraine, headaches, high blood pressure caused by nervousness, high blood cholesterol, arteriosclerosis, and diarrhoea.

Pellagra. Niacin's greatest claim to fame lies in the prevention and cure of pellagra. Early symptoms of this disease, such as loss of appetite and weight, followed by general weakness, are relieved quickly. Symptoms like a sore mouth, digestive and nervous disturbances, skin eruptions, particularly on the hands, arms, feet, and legs, take longer to heal. Even the administration of small amounts of niacin of upto 10 mg or 10,000 mcg per day is sufficient to cure endemic pellagra.

Migraine. Niacin has been found useful in treating migraines. Persons suffering from migraine and high blood pressure brought on by nervousness, are said to get tremendous relief by taking large doses of niacin.

Heart-Related Disorders. Niacin has been found to provide relief in angina pectoris. It has also been found useful in cases of cerebral thrombosis, caused by blockage of the blood vessels of the brain due to clots of blood. Instances of blood clots in the brain caused by rupturing of cerebral arteries were first reported cleared up with niacin by Dr Diego Furtado of the University of Lisbon in Portugal.

High Blood Pressure. Niacin has been used as a vasodilator to dilate blood vessels and to correct blood pressure changes. It is said to be particularly effective in preventing and relieving high blood pressure caused by nervousness.

High Blood Cholesterol. Niacin has proved to have a remarkable effect in reducing high blood cholesterol. In a study conducted by D. G. Moore Fitzgerald of St. Vincent's Hospital, Dublin, it was reported that in patients who had more than 530 mg of blood cholesterol, a remarkable fall touching 230 mg of blood cholesterol was attained on continuous administration of 3 g of niacin daily, in three divided doses.

Diarrhoea. It has been found that diarrhoea can result from a variety of nutritional deficiencies, particularly a lack of niacin. The administration of this vitamin in therapeutic doses along with other B vitamins can cure such ailments.

Precautions. The use of large doses of niacin for long periods causes release of histamine. This in turn can cause severe flushing, severe itching of the skin(pruritis), and gastro-intestinal disturbances.

If taken in doses of 3 g per day, niacin has been reported to cause elevation of uric acid in the blood and glucose.

The Anti-Stress Factor

Vitamin B_5 is a water-soluble vitamin of the B complex group. Also known as pantothenic acid, it was discovered in 1933 by Roger Williams. Tissue extracts from a variety of biological materials

Recommended Daily Allowance	
Men	10 mg
Women	10 mg
Children	5.5 mg

provided a growth factor for yeast. This growth factor was identified as pantothenic acid, derived from the Greek word *pantos*, meaning 'everywhere'. It was first recognised as essential for rats, dogs, pigs, pigeons, and chicks. Williams isolated this vitamin in 1939 and later synthesised it(prepared it through chemical processes).

Pantothenic acid is a pale yellow, oily liquid which is not crystallised, but its calcium salt crystallises readily and this is the form in which it is generally available. This vitamin is not destroyed in neutral solutions, but is liable to rapid destruction in acid and alkaline mediums. It is also liable to destruction by food-processing techniques, caffeine, sulphur drugs, sleeping pills, and alcohol. Pantothenic acid is absorbed from the alimentary tract, and excreted in urine and mother's milk.

Functions in the Body

Pantothenic acid is a part of the enzyme system which plays a vital role in the metabolism of carbohydrates, fats, and proteins, and in the synthesis of amino acids and fatty acids. It is also essential for the formation of porphyrin, the pigment portion of the haemoglobin molecule of the red blood cells.

This vitamin is involved in all the vital functions of the body. It stimulates the adrenal glands and increases production of cortisone and other adrenal hormones. It is primarily used as an anti-stress factor and protects against most physical and mental stresses and toxins. Pantothenic acid increases vitality, wards off infections, and speeds recovery from ill health. It helps in maintaining the normal growth and development of the central nervous system. This vitamin prevents premature ageing. It also provides protection against any damage caused by excessive radiation.

Sources

Pantothenic acid is found in extensive quantities in foods. The best sources are yeast, liver, and eggs. Other good sources are peanuts, mushrooms, split peas, soya beans and soya bean flour. About one-half of the pantothenic acid is lost in the milling of grains. Fruits are relatively poor sources of this vitamin.

Rich Sources of Vitamin B₅(Pantothenic Acid)*

Cereals	mcg	Vegetables	mcg
Oatmeal, dry	1,500	Mushrooms	2,200
Wheat germ, toasted	1,200	Broccoli	1,200
Brown rice	1,100	Cauliflower	1,000
Wheat flour, whole	1,100	**Nuts & Oilseeds**	
Pulses & Legumes		Peanuts	2,800
Soya bean flour	2,000	Sunflower seeds	1,400
Split peas	2,000	Cashew nuts	1,300
Soya beans	1,700	**Meat**	
Lentil	1,400	Liver, calf	8,000
Blackeye peas, dry	1,000		

* Values per 100 g edible portions.

Deficiency Symptoms

A deficiency of pantothenic acid can cause chronic fatigue, an increased tendency towards infections, greying and loss of hair, mental depression, irritability, dizziness, and muscular weakness. It may lead to stomach distress, constipation, skin disorders, retarded growth, painful and burning feet, insomnia, muscle cramps, exhaustion, low blood sugar, low blood pressure, and duodenal ulcers.

Healing and Therapeutic Properties

The usual therapeutic doses of pantothenic acid are 50-200 mg. In some studies 1,000 mg and more were given daily for six months without any side-effects being produced.

Stress. The use of pantothenic acid has been found valuable in meeting the demands of stress. In one study, the effect of large quantities of patothenic acid was tested on healthy men suffering from stress. These volunteers were immersed in cold water for eight minutes before being given this vitamin, and eight minutes again after receiving 10,000 mg of calcium pantothenate daily for six weeks. Their stress lasted only for eight minutes, yet the pantothenic acid prevented destruction of protein, retention of salt, and a rise in blood sugar. It caused the blood cholesterol to fall. There were no toxic effects.

Arthritis. The use of pantothenic acid is considered valuable in arthritis. Dr E. C. Barton-Wright, a microbiologist, believed that arthritis was a vitamin-deficiency disease which could be prevented or relieved by a diet containing adequate amounts of pantothenic acid. Dr W. A. Eliot and Dr Barton-Wright (both from UK) were the first to show that the pantothenic acid content of the blood of persons suffering from rheumatoid arthritis was lower than that in healthy individuals. In some cases, 1,000 mg administered daily was found effective in reducing the pain caused by arthritis.

Infections. Pantothenic acid plays an important role in the body during infections by protecting the liver. While treating infections with antibiotics, the addition of pantothenic acid also minimises the chances of drug-resistant organisms, reduces the risk of untoward reactions to the antibiotics, and increases antibodies in the body.

Skin Disorders. Administration of pantothenic acid either orally or by injection, or by external application in the form of ointment or solution, is helpful for sunburn and old-age dermatitis.

Premature Greying. Pantothenic acid is one of the three anti-grey-hair vitamins, the other two being para-aminobenzoic acid and inositol. Many people with grey hair have taken pantothenic acid and some have had their hair restored to their natural colour. However, for satisfactory results, all the three anti-grey-hair vitamins should be taken simultaneously, preferably in a form which provides all the B vitamins, such as yeast, wheat germ, and liver.

The 'Versatile' Vitamin

In 1926, J. Goldberger and R. D. Lillie fed rats on a diet deficient in what was considered to be the pellagra-preventive factor. These animals developed dermatitis. P. Gyorgy later observed that the

Recommended Daily Allowance	
Men	2.0 mg
Women	2.0 mg
Children	1.7 mg
Infants	0.1-0.4 mg

same factor prevented the development of skin lesion in rats. He proposed that this factor be called vitamin B_6. Goldberger's pellagra-preventive factor, riboflavin, and vitamin B_6 were shown to be different substances.

Vitamin B_6 was isolated in 1938 by three research groups working independently and was synthesised by S. A. Harris and K. Folkers in 1939.

Vitamin B_6 is a white, crystalline substance. It is soluble in water and alcohol. Long storage, canning, roasting or stewing of meat, food-processing techniques, use of alcohol, and oestrogen are destructive to this vitamin.

Vitamin B_6 is absorbed mainly in the jejunum. However it is also absorbed in the ileum of the small intestine by passive diffusion. Absorption in the colon is very slight. Although the bacteria in the colon do synthesise vitamin B_6, it is not absorbed to any significant extent. Small quantities of this vitamin are stored in the body. The vitamin is widely distributed in various tissues and excreted mainly from the kidneys. Small quantities of the vitamin are excreted in the faeces and in sweat.

Functions in the Body

Pyridoxine aids in food assimilation and protein and fat metabolism, especially in the metabolism of essential fatty acids. It activates many enzymes and enzyme systems. It is involved in the production of antibodies which protect against bacterial diseases. Pyridoxine helps in the healthy functioning of the nervous system and brain. It is essential for the normal reproductive process and healthy pregnancies.

This vitamin prevents nervous and skin disorders, provides protection against a high cholesterol level, certain types of heart disease, and diabetes. It prevents tooth decay. Vitamin B_6 regulates the balance between sodium and potassium in the body, which is vitally important for normal body functions. It is also required for absorption of vitamin B_{12} and for the production of hydrochloric acid and magnesium.

Sources

Yeast, sunflower seeds, wheat germ, soya beans, and walnuts are the richest sources of pyridoxine among plant foods. Lentils, lima beans, and other vegetables provide fair amounts. Raw foods contain more of this vitamin than cooked foods.

Deficiency Symptoms

Deficiency of vitamin B_6 may cause anaemia, oedema, mental depression, and skin disorders. Cracking at the corner of the lips, halitosis(foul smell in the mouth), nervousness, eczema, kidney stones, inflammation of the colon, damage to the pancreas, insomnia, tooth decay, and irritability may also result due to deficiency of vitamin B_6. Inadequate intake of the vitamin may also lead to loss of muscular control, migraine headaches, diseases of old age, and premature senility.

Rich Sources of Vitamin B₆ (Pyridoxine)*

Cereals	mcg		mcg
Wheat germ, toasted	1,150	Potatoes	250
Brown rice	550	Cauliflower	200
Wheat flour, whole	350	Sweet potatoes	200
Barley	200	**Nuts & Oilseeds**	
Pulses & Legumes		Sunflower seeds	1,250
Soya beans, dry	800	Walnuts	750
Soya bean flour	650	Chestnuts, fresh	350
Lentil, dry	600	**Fruits**	
Lima beans, dry	600	Bananas	500
Vegetables		Avocados	400
Spinach	300	Prunes	250
Brussels sprouts	250	Raisins	250

* Values per 100 g edible portions.

Healing and Therapeutic Properties

Vitamin B_6 is now being considered as a wonder treatment for a wide range of common ailments.

Diabetes. Vitamin B_6 has been found beneficial in the treatment of diabetes. All diabetics appear to excrete a large amount of xanthurenic acid, which is indicative of vitamin B_6 deficiency. Experiments have shown that there is a rapid drop in the urinary excretion of this acid when 50 mg of vitamin B_6 is given daily to patients suffering from diabetes.

Haemorrhoids. Vitamin B_6 has proved to be valuable in curing haemorrhoids. Experiments were conducted on volunteers deficient in vitamin B_6 and they were found to be suffering from bleeding haemorrhoids. On being given therapeutic doses of this vitamin, the haemorrhoids disappeared. Rapid recovery has been reported in several cases of this disease when 10 mg of vitamin B_6 has been given after each meal as a supplement. As pregnant women are generally deficient in vitamin B_6, a lack of this vitamin may be the cause of haemorrhoids which are commonly prevalent during this period.

Convulsions in Infants and Women. Infants who are fed on powdered milk are generally found to be deficient in vitamin B_6. This deficiency causes convulsions without fever. Administration of 0.5 to 10 mg of vitamin B_6, three times daily, relieves convulsions.

It has also been found that during pregnancy, undernourished women usually lack in vitamin B_6 due to an excessive demand by the foetus. This deficiency affects the development of the central nervous system of the foetus. This causes demylination(uncovering of the nerve fibres of the peripheral nerves), resulting in epileptic-like seizures. In all such conditions where there is no other apparent or known cause of convulsions, administering 50 mg of vitamin B_6, three times daily, is found to be a very effective treatment.

Vaginal Bleeding. Long-standing irregular vaginal bleeding in young girls can be successfully treated with vitamin B_6. Vitamin B_6 controls the bleeding by inhibiting the activity of oestrogen and the ripening of the follicles.

Stress and Insomnia. On account of its sedative action on the central nervous system, the use of vitamin B_6 has been found to be of valuable assistance in psychoneurosis, mental irritability, general weakness, sleeplessness, and mental stress. In all these conditions, vitamin B_6 should be administered in doses of 40 mg, three times daily.

Morning Sickness and Travel Sickness. The use of vitamin B_6 has been found beneficial in the treatment of morning sickness during pregnancy. Its sedative action reduces travel sickness too. To achieve gratifying results this vitamin can be given in doses of 40 mg early in the morning during pregnancy, and an hour before travelling. The dose can be repeated once every four hours if the sick feeling persists.

Precautions. The toxicity of all forms of vitamin B_6 is low. However that does not mean that vitamin B_6 can be taken at random. Heavy doses of vitamin B_6 should not be taken unless the individual has been found to have a deficiency. The progress of patients taking such heavy doses should be carefully monitored. A possible symptom of an over-dosage of vitamin B_6 is night restlessness.

Strengthens Immunity

Biotin(vitamin B_8) is a member of the B complex group. In 1927, M. A. Boas made the important discovery that when the egg-white of a raw egg was administered as the main source of protein in the

Recommended Daily Allowance	
Men	100-200 mcg
Women	100-200 mcg
Children	50-200 mcg
Infants	35 mcg

diets of rats, they developed deficiency symptoms characterised by dermatitis, loss of hair, and muscular incoordination. All these symptoms were prevented or cured by yeast, liver, and egg yolk. The factor was called 'anti-egg-white injury factor'. In 1931, Gyorgy gave the name Vitamin H to this factor(Hant in German means skin). It was isolated in 1939 by P. Gyorgy, R. Kuhn, and Lederer and was called biotin.

Biotin is one of the most active biological substances known. An extremely small amount of this vitamin has a marked effect on the growth of yeast and certain bacteria. It forms part of several enzyme systems. Biotin is freely soluble in hot water, but sparingly in cold water. It is insoluble in fat solvents and sparingly soluble in alcohol. Water, sulpha drugs, oestrogen, food processing techniques, alcohol, and, in particular, large quantities of egg white can destroy this vitamin.

Functions in the Body

Biotin is vital for a healthy immune system. It is involved in the metabolism of corbohydrates, proteins, and fats. It is essential for the growth and health of the hair. It prevents premature greying of the hair as well as hair loss. This vitamin helps to maintain the skin and the nervous system in a sound condition. It controls proper distribution of colour pigment.

Sources

The rich sources of biotin are brewer's yeast, beef liver, rice bran, rice germ, rice polishings, and peanut butter. This vitamin is also normally produced in the intestines if there are a sufficient amount of healthy intestinal flora present. However, frequent use of antibiotics can interfere with the synthesis of this vitamin.

Rich Sources of Biotin*

Cereals	mcg		mcg
Rice bran	60	Split peas	20
Rice polishings	60	Lentil	10
Rice germ	40	**Vegetables**	
Barley	30	Mushrooms	15
Oatmeal	25	Cauliflower	15
Whole wheat	15		
Brown rice	10	**Nuts**	
Pulses & Legumes		Walnuts	40
		Peanuts, roasted	35
Soya bean flour	70	Almonds	20
Soya beans	60	**Meat**	
Blackeye peas	20	Beef liver	100

* Values per 100 g edible portions.

Deficiency Symptoms

Since it is of great importance in human nutrition, deficiency of biotin causes muscular weakness, pains, pins and needles(pricking of the skin), lassitude, and lack of appetite. It may cause eczema, dandruff, hair loss, and seborrhoea. Other common problems which may occur are skin disorders, heart abnormalities, lung infections, anaemia, extreme fatigue, confusion, mental depression, and drowsiness. The fleshy part of the tongue may waste away.

Healing and Therapeutic Properties

Treatment with 20 mcg of biotin, taken daily for 10 days intramuscularly, can heal skin lesions in about 90 per cent of infants with seborrheic dermatitis. Oral biotin taken in amounts of 400 mcg daily for 8–12 weeks, or 600 mcg taken daily for 6-8 weeks, has been used with good success in the treatment of acne and seborrheic eczema. The use of a tropical creamy preparation once daily, and a shampoo containing 0.25-1.0 per cent biotin, three times weekly, has been found effective in reducing and controlling excessive hair loss in male alopecia.

VITAMIN B_9 — FOLIC ACID

Prevents Anaemia

Vitamin B_9 or folic acid, also known as folacin and folate, was first recognised as a dietary essential for chicks in 1938. Later it was found to be essential for other animals and human beings too. It was used clinically in 1945 by T. D. Spies, who found it to be

Recommended Daily Allowance	
Men	100 mcg
Women	100 mcg
Preg. Wo.*	400 mcg
Lact. Wo**	150 mcg
Children	80 mcg
Infants	25 mcg

effective in the treatment of anaemias relating to pregnancy and tropical sprue(an intestinal malabsorption condition). These findings were subsequently confirmed.

Folic acid is a yellow, crystalline substance, sparingly soluble in water and stable in acid solution. However it undergoes fairly rapid destruction when heated in neutral or alkaline substances. It may thus be destroyed by some methods of cooking. Factors that damage this vitamin are sulphur drugs, sunlight, and food processing.

Folic acid is absorbed along the entire length of the intestine, although the jejunum of the small intestine is the primary site for its absorption. About half of the folic acid stored in the body is in the liver which contains 5 to 15 mg/kg of liver weight. A small amount is excreted in the faeces and urine but the additional amounts are presumed to be

---

* Preg. Wo. — Pregnant Women.

** Lact. Wo. — Lactating Women.

metabolised and also lost by cells coming off in scales from body surfaces.

Functions in the Body

Folic acid, in combination with vitamin B_{12}, is essential for the formation, maturation and multiplication of red blood cells. It is necessary for the growth and division of all body cells, including nerve cells, and for manufacturing a number of nerve transmitters. It also produces nucleic acids, RNA(ribonucleic acid) and DNA(deoxyribonucleic acid), that carry hereditary patterns. It aids in protein metabolism and contributes to normal growth. Folic acid helps in the building of antibodies which prevent and heal infections. It is essential for the health of the skin and hair, and helps to prevent premature greying of the hair.

Folic acid is the singlemost important nutrient for a pregnant woman and her developing foetus. In fact, eating fresh fruits and vegetables rich in folate, from conception until the due date, is the best policy a woman can adopt to ensure that her pregnancy will be a happy and a healthy one. Folic acid also improves lactation.

Sources

Pulses and legumes such as Bengal gram and green gram are rich in folic acid. Green vegetables such as amaranth, cluster beans, spinach, and mint are valuable sources of folic acid. In fact, the presence of this vitamin in green leaves was the basis for the name folacin(*folium* meaning leaf). Besides green leaves, folic acid is found in gingelly seeds, and meat.

Deficiency Symptoms

Deficiency of folic acid causes anaemia which often occurs in pregnant women and children. Serious skin

Rich Sources of Vitamin B₉ (Folic Acid)*

Cereals	mcg		mcg
Bajra	14.7	Cluster beans	50.0
Jowar	14.0	Amaranth, tender,	
Maize, dry	14.0	gangeticus	41.0
Wheat flour, whole	12.1	Ladies' fingers	25.3
		Curry leaves	23.5
Pulses & Legumes		Colocasia	16.0
Cowpeas	69.0	French beans	15.5
Bengal gram, whole	34.0		
Split Bengal gram	32.0	**Nuts & Oilseeds**	
Split green gram	24.5	Gingelly seeds	51.0
Split black gram	24.0	Groundnuts	16.0
Bengal gram, roasted	22.0	Coconut, dry	15.3
Split red gram	19.0		
Lentil	14.5	**Meat & Poultry**	
		Eggs	70.3
Vegetables		Liver, sheep	65.5
Spinach	51.0	Liver, goat	61.2

* Values per 100 g edible portions.

---

disorders, loss of hair, impaired circulation, a greyish-brown skin pigmentation, fatigue, and mental depression can result from a deficiency of this vitamin. Reproductive disorders such as spontaneous abortions and difficult labour, and a high infant death rate can also be caused by folic acid deficiency. Vitamin B₉ deficiency may also lead to loss of libido in males. According to studies, two-thirds of geriatric patients were found to be deficient in folic acid, while one-third of psychiatric patients were also deficient in this vitamin. Lack of folic acid can also lead to dementia.

Almost all the anticonvulsant drugs used in the treatment of epilepsy reduce serum folate concentrations. In addition to anticonvulsants, other drugs such as oral contraceptives, pyrimethamine (an antimalarial), co-trim-oxazole (contains a sulphur compound), and ethanol (alcohol) may impair folate metabolism.

Healing and Therapeutic Properties

Large doses of folic acid have been found beneficial in the treatment of a few diseases which are rare and often involve mental retardation. Some of these diseases were detected initially by the presence of megaloblastic anaemia, a state suggestive of defective folic acid metabolism.

Megaloblastic Anaemia. Folic acid is required for the treatment of nutritional megaloblastic anaemia during pregnancy and infancy. A daily dose of 5,000 to 10,000 mcg taken orally is usually sufficient. It is also advisable to take a small daily dose(around 400 mcg) of this vitamin during pregnancy. The Food and Drug Association of America(FDA) has also approved the claim that folic acid supplements can prevent certain birth defects.

Sprue. Folic acid has been found valuable in curing sprue, an intestinal disease characterised by a sore mouth and tongue, anaemia, severe diarrhoea, and large amounts of fat in the stools. This disease results from deficiency of folic acid and can be remedied by daily injections of 25 mg or 25,000 mcg of this vitamin. As food is poorly absorbed in this condition, a diet containing even sixty times that amount does not bring improvement. With the injection, however, improvement can be noticed in a single day and within a few days, the patient can absorb the vitamin well orally. Ultimately the diet for sprue must make up for the multiple and severe deficiencies resulting from diarrhoea.

Recurrent Abortion. Folic acid has proved beneficial in the treatment of recurrent abortions. It is, therefore, advisable to take 10,000 mcg of folic acid daily, with iron and B_{12}, from the beginning of pregnancy till its completion.

Mental Retardation. Folic acid supplements have been used to improve the mental function and the quality of life among mentally retarded children. In the case of epileptic children and mentally deranged persons, regular treatment with 5,000 mcg of folic acid, three times daily, gets a quick healing response, and in many individuals, there has been a complete resolution of mental symptoms.

Brown Spots on the Skin. Deficiency of folic acid, associated with vitamin B_{12} deficiency, causes darkish brown spotty pigmentation that usually appears on the face, inner mouth, under the arm pits, over the thighs, and on the palms. This happens particularly in the case of pregnant women and women on the pill. In such cases, administration of 10 mg or 10,000 mcg of folic acid, along with 100 mcg of vitamin B_{12}, taken thrice daily, shows a remarkable amelioration of the brownish pigmentation.

Gout. Though most cases of gout are treated with dietary therapy, if additional support is necessary, folic acid is recommended in the range of 10-40 mg per day.

Precautions. Folic acid normally has no adverse effects. However, when it is used to treat megaloblastic anaemia(secondary to the use of anticonvulsant drugs), the epilepsy may be aggravated. If prescribed in the treatment of gout, it may interfere with drugs being prescribed for epilepsy, and hide the symptoms of a vitamin B_{12} deficiency. Hence folic acid therapy in gout too should only be taken under medical supervision.

VITAMIN B$_{12}$ — CYANOCOBALAMIN

Stimulates Growth of Red Blood Cells

In 1948 two independent groups of workers led by E. L. Smith in Great Britain and L. F. Parker in USA isolated vitamin B$_{12}$ from the liver. Hodgkin, the 1964 Nobel Prize winner for

Recommended Daily Allowance		
Men	1	mcg
Women	1	mcg
Children	0.2-1	mcg
Infants	0.2	mcg

chemistry, and her co-workers delineated the structural formula of vitamin B$_{12}$. They concluded that this vitamin was produced only by fungi and bacteria. Human intestinal bacteria also produced appreciable quantities of it. It was effective in a type of anaemia called pernicious anaemia, in as small a quantity as one-millionth part of a gram. Its deficiency in the body occurred usually due to malabsorption from the intestine rather than from malnutrition.

Vitamin B$_{12}$ is freely soluble in water. It is resistant to boiling in neutral solutions, but is liable to destruction in the presence of alkalies and acids. Other factors that destroy this vitamin are sunlight, alcohol, oestrogen — the female hormone, and sleeping pills.

Deficiency of vitamin B$_{12}$ is caused more frequently by problems of absorption than by dietary inadequacy. The presence of a sufficient quantity of gastric juice is essential to facilitate its absorption in the intestine. Calcium and protein-rich food greatly help the absorption of this vitamin from the intestines. The amount of vitamin B$_{12}$ which is not immediately needed by the body is stored in the liver, which is capable of storing relatively large amounts of this nutrient.

About 30 mcg of vitamin B_{12} are excreted in the normal urine daily. When injected in a large dose upto 100 mcg, upto 90 per cent of the quantity is excreted. Since the absorption of vitamin B_{12} does not take place in the colon, much of the unabsorbed vitamin B_{12} is excreted in the stools. This vitamin is also secreted in breast milk for the use of babies.

Functions in the Body

Like vitamin B_6, vitamin B_{12} is essential for the production and regeneration of red blood cells. It is also needed for the proper functioning of the central nervous system. It improves concentration, memory, and balance, and relieves irritability. Vitamin B_{12} is necessary for proper utilisation of fats, carbohydrates, and proteins for body building. It promotes growth and increases appetite in children. This vitamin is also involved in many vital metabolic and enzymatic processes, including the metabolism of folic acid. If the immune cells made in the bone marrow are to mature into active disease-fighters, a sufficient quantity of vitamin B_{12} and folic acid are necessary.

Sources

Vitamin B_{12} is unique amongst vitamins in that it is mostly found in foods of animal origin. Meat, liver, eggs, shrimps, and dairy products are valuable sources of this vitamin. Vegetarians are therefore advised to increase their intake of milk or take vitamin B_{12} in a tablet form as a supplement.

Deficiency Symptoms

A deficiency of vitamin B_{12} may cause pernicious (destructive) anaemia. It may lead to a poor appetite and retardation of growth in children, chronic fatigue,

Rich Sources of Vitamin B$_{12}$ (Cyanocobalamin)*

Fish, Meat & Poultry	mcg	Milk & Milk Products	mcg
Liver, sheep	91.9	Skimmed milk	
Liver, goat	90.4	powder	0.83
Shrimps, fresh	9.0	Milk, buffalo's	0.14
Egg, yolk	4.4	Milk, cow's	0.14
Goat meat	2.8	Curd, cow's milk	0.13
Mutton	2.6	Curd, buffalo's milk	0.10
Eggs, whole	1.8		
Buffalo meat	1.7		

* Values per 100 g edible portions.

a sore mouth, a feeling of numbness or stiffness, loss of mental energy, and difficulty in concentration.

Deficiency of vitamin B$_{12}$ affects every cell in the body, but is most severely felt in the tissues where the cells normally divide rapidly, as in the blood-forming tissues of the bone marrow and in the gastro-intestinal tract. The nervous system is also affected and this may lead to degeneration of nerve fibres in the spinal cord and peripheral nerves.

Healing and Therapeutic Properties

Vitamin B$_{12}$ is administered orally in doses from 6 to 150 mcg. Taken in these doses, it helps in the treatment of lack of concentration, fatigue, depression, insomnia, anorexia, loss of weight due to deficiency of this vitamin, and poor memory. As this vitamin is difficult to assimilate when taken orally, most doctors administer it in the form of injections ranging from 100-1,000 mcg if used for therapeutic purposes.

Anaemia. Given by injection, this vitamin provides complete and satisfactory treatment in cases of pernicious anaemia. The general practice is to give 1,000 mcg of vitamin B$_{12}$ by injection, twice weekly, until the haemoglobin level is restored to normal. Subsequently an injection of 1,000 mcg every six weeks is all that is needed to keep the patient in good health. These doses may appear to be excessive since much of the vitamin is excreted in the urine. Nevertheless it is not unreasonable to give large doses at first to refill the depleted reserves.

A similar dose schedule is required in cases of sub-acute combined degeneration of the cord, a disorder of the spinal cord which affects the conduction of nerve impulses.

Smoking. Studies show that smokers have lower levels of vitamin B_{12} and folic acid than non-smokers. Seventy-three longtime smokers with precancerous cell changes in their lung secretions, were taken as case studies. Half were given B_{12} and folic acid supplements for four months; the other half were given placebos(inactive substances). After four months, a recheck of the lung fluids showed that those who were given vitamin therapy showed less precancerous changes than those who were administered placebos.

Precautions. There are no known toxic effects of vitamin B_{12} even when it is taken in mega doses.

For a Healthy Liver

Choline is a member of the vitamin B group. Its importance in nutrition was established by C. H. Best and M. E. Huntsman in 1934. They discovered that choline deficiency produced a fatty liver.

Recommended Daily Allowance		
Men	1,000	mg
Women	1,000	mg
Children	550	mg

Choline is present in foods as well as in the body in relatively large amounts. The body can make choline from methionine(see pages 177 to 178), an amino acid, with the aid of vitamin B_{12} and folic acid.

Choline is a colourless, crystalline compound which absorbs water quickly. It is highly soluble in water and alcohol. Dilute solutions of choline(less than 4 per cent) are not destroyed by heat. However, when concentrated solutions of choline are boiled, it decomposes. Choline is also destroyed by water, sulphur drugs, food-processing techniques, and alcohol. Choline is absorbed from the intestine and excreted mostly through the urine.

Functions in the Body

Choline helps in the transportation of fats in the body and prevents accumulation of fat in the liver. This vitamin works with inositol, another vitamin of the B group, to utilise fats and cholesterol. In combination with fatty acids and phosphorus, it stimulates the formation of lecithin, an important constituent of nerve cells in the body. Choline is one of the few substances which penetrates the so-called blood-brain barrier, which ordinarily protects the brain against the effects

65

of variations in the daily diet. It goes directly into the brain cells to produce a chemical that aids memory.

Sources

Choline is available in liberal quantities in fish and sea foods.

Rich Sources of Choline*

Cereals, Pulses & Legumes	mg	Nuts & Oilseeds	mg
		Groundnuts	224
French millet	748	Mustard seeds	211
Field beans, dry	352	**Fruits**	
Lentil	299	Apples	321
Peas, dry	235	Indian gooseberries	256
Split black gram	206	**Fish & Sea Food**	
Wheat, bulgar	206	Indian shard	1,364
Cowpeas	202	Folui	1,018
Bengal gram, whole	194	*Pabda*	1,018
Split red gram	183	*Chital*	943
Green gram, whole	167	Pangas	913
		Koi	891
Vegetables		Rohu	819
Beetroot	242	*Tengra,* fresh	783
Lettuce	178	Kalabasu	716
Carrots	168	Magur	639
Turnips	137	Katla	611
Pumpkin	136	Sole	572
Cauliflower	127	Prawns	542
Cabbage	120	Mrigal	480
Potatoes	100	*Bam*	438
Radishes, white	63	*Puti*	393

* Values per 100 g edible portions.

Deficiency Symptoms

A prolonged deficiency of choline may cause cirrhosis and the fatty degeneration of the liver, high blood pressure, and atherosclerosis(hardening of the arteries).

Healing and Therapeutic Properties

Oral administration of choline, as well as lecithin, has been found to be effective in increasing serum choline levels in human beings.

Nephritis. Choline has been found beneficial in the treatment of nephritis(inflammation of the kidneys). Addition of choline to an otherwise adequate diet has quickly corrected experimentally produced nephritis in laboratory animals. Calves receiving no choline died within seven days of severe haemorrhaging nephritis. Other calves kept on the same diet, but given 1,000 mg of choline, made noticeable improvement within 24 hours. The experimentally produced nephritis was found to be similar to the disease seen in man. In an experiment, 51 out of 102 people with fatty livers, recognised as choline deficiency, had high blood urea and albumin in the urine, showing mild nephritis. This disease quickly disappeared when choline was given with an adequate diet. Giving choline with inositol or lecithin, however, is much more effective than choline alone.

Liver Damage. The effect of choline has been widely studied in different laboratory animals. In rats deficient in choline, it has been observed that fat accumulates in the liver cells within a few hours. In a short time, they become swollen with fat. Consequently, many of these cells may actually burst. The fat combines into pools and seeps into the blood and bile. Unless choline is added to the diet, scars replace most of the liver tissue, a condition similar to human cirrhosis, which is fatal to animals and humans alike. However, the liver again becomes healthy if choline is given early enough.

High Blood Pressure. High blood pressure has been repeatedly produced in animals on diets deficient in choline. In an experiment, 158 patients with severe hypertension were studied while being given choline daily. All the patients had been on various medications for a year or longer without improvement. All medication was discontinued before they were given choline. Such symptoms as headaches, dizziness, noises in the ear, palpitations, and constipation improved or disappeared completely in five to ten days after the vitamin was started. The blood pressure began to fall within three weeks and decreased in every case, the average drop being 31 mm systolic and 20 mm diastolic. In more than one-third of these patients, the blood pressure dropped to normal, but not below normal. Insomnia, trembling, swelling of the body, and visual disturbances were gradually relieved.

Heart Disease. Choline, along with inositol, has been found beneficial in the treatment of heart disease. Patients recovering from heart attacks showed a decrease in the size of cholesterol particles and the amount of fat in the blood when given 2,000 and 750 mg of choline and inositol, respectively. Two months later, their blood cholesterol became normal and blood lecithin also increased. When choline was given alone, the cholesterol was reduced.

Precautions. Oral administration of large quantities of choline and lecithin produces adverse side-effects, including diarrhoea, nausea, salivation, and depression.

Prevents Hair Loss

Inositol is a member of the vitamin B group. It is a crystalline compound which has a sweet taste. It is highly soluble in water, and is not destroyed by heat in neutral, acid, and alkaline mediums. It is,

Recommended Daily Allowance		
Men	1,000	mg
Women	1,000	mg
Children	550	mg

however, destroyed by sulphur drugs, food-processing techniques, alcohol, and coffee.

Over 99 per cent of ingested inositol is absorbed by the body. However, absorption is slow. It is catabolised in the kidneys, where it is converted to glucose.

Functions in the Body

Inositol is essential for the transportation of fat in the body. Like choline, it has been found important in providing nourishment to the brain cells. It helps lower cholesterol levels. Inositol also promotes the growth of healthy hair and helps to prevent its falling. It helps in preventing eczema.

Sources

The most important sources of inositol are liver, brewer's yeast, dried lima beans, beef brain and heart, grapefruit, raisins, wheat germ, unrefined molasses, peanuts, and cabbage.

Deficiency Symptoms

According to R. A. McCance and E. M. Widdowson, the deficiency of inositol can cause alopecia or patchy baldness, gastritis, hypertension, fatty infiltration in the liver, hardening of the liver, and eczema.

Healing and Therapeutic Properties

Therapeutic administration of inositol in quantities of 2 g a day, for 6-10 weeks, has resulted in small reductions in plasma cholesterol levels in hypercholesterolemic patients.

Premature Greying. Inositol is one of the three anti-grey-hair B group vitamins, the other two being pantothenic acid and para-aminobenzoic acid (paba). A liberal intake of inositol of upto 2,000 mg, along with 10 mg of pantothenic acid, and 100 mg of paba, usually changes grey hair back to its normal colour. It would be preferable to take all these three vitamins in a form which provides all the vitamins of the B group such as yeast, wheat germ, and liver.

Baldness. Bald-headedness in men is considered to be a partly nutritional deficiency caused by lack of inositol. A deficiency of this vitamin causes animals to lose their hair. When inositol is added to their diet again, a new and healthy coat of hair grows. Interestingly enough, male animals lose their hair in half the time that female animals do. Concentrated inositol has been used in a few cases of bald-headedness with promising results. New growth has been seen within two months, and healthy hair of a natural colour slowly fills the gap from the back forwards, and around the edges of the bald spot, toward the centre. Research indicates that women have a low requirement of inositol. Although this vitamin may help to stimulate the growth of a woman's hair, its lack is probably not a major cause of slow growth.

Heart Disease. Inositol, along with choline, has been found valuable in the treatment of heart disease(*see Choline*).

The 'Antibiotic' Vitamin

The story of vitamin C or ascorbic acid is most interesting and fascinating. In the 18th century, a British naval surgeon, James Lind, demonstrated that the juices of citrus fruits like oranges, limes, and lemons prevented and cured

Recommended Daily Allowance		
Men	40	mg
Women	40	mg
Lact. Wo.	80	mg
Children	40	mg
Infants	25	mg

scurvy, a disease characterised by bleeding from the gums and other parts of the body after or without an injury. This disease was widely prevalent among sailors on long voyages as they had to subsist on salt, fish, meat, and bread, and were entirely deprived of any fresh food.

It was, however, only in 1928 that vitamin C was isolated. In that year, Szent Gyrogyi, while working in Hopkin's laboratory, isolated ascorbic acid from different sources such as the suprarenal glands in the body, and fruits and vegetables like oranges and cabbage. However he did not recognise its properties as a vitamin. Thereafter, in 1932, another of Hopkin's students, Glen King, isolated the vitamin from lemon juice and identified it with Szent Gyrogyi's acid. Within a few months, W. N. Haworth and E. L. Hirst in Birmingham, elucidated the chemical structure of ascorbic acid and accomplished its synthesis. In 1938 'ascorbic acid' was officially accepted as the chemical name for vitamin C.

Vitamin C appears in a white crystal form and is readily soluble in water. This vitamin is easily destroyed by heat, oxidation, drying, and storage. Alkalinity, even to a slight degree, is distinctly destructive to this vitamin. Acid fruits and vegetables lose much less ascorbic acid on heating than non-acid foods. This vitamin is lost from some vegetables during the first few minutes of cooking.

Absorption of ascorbic acid into the bloodstream takes place in the upper part of the small intestine. The amount of ascorbic acid in different tissues varies: the adrenal and pituitary tissue, brain, pancreas, kidneys, liver, and spleen have relatively high concentrations; blood cells contain even more than the bloodstream.

Vitamin C is excreted by the kidneys through the urine. Excretion is diminished or absent when the body is already depleted of it. When there is an intake of over 3 g of vitamin C per day, the unabsorbed ascorbic acid is largely excreted in the faeces, and to a smaller extent, in the urine.

Functions in the Body

One of the most significant functions of vitamin C is the formation of collagen, a protein substance that cements the cells together. Failure to synthesise collagen results in delayed healing of wounds.

Ascorbic acid enhances the absorption of iron. It is needed for buoyant health, vitality, and endurance. It ensures a clear skin, a fresh complexion, and healthy gums and teeth. It is involved in the vital functions of all glands and organs. This vitamin is also necessary for maintenance of bones and proper functioning of the adrenal and thyroid glands. It promotes healing and protects against all forms of stress — physical and mental. It also provides protection against the harmful effects of toxic chemicals in the environment, food, and water, and counteracts the toxic effect of drugs.

Sources

The main sources of vitamin C are citrus fruits and vegetables. Among fruits, Indian gooseberries, guavas, limes, lemons, oranges, and papayas are the most valuable sources of this vitamin. Root vegetables and potatoes contain smaller amounts. Potatoes, however, account for a large proportion of the total ascorbic acid intake because of the amount normally eaten every day. Foodstuffs of animal origin contain only small amounts of this vitamin; the more important of such sources is fish. Cereals and pulses do not contain vitamin C in the dry state, but if soaked in water for about 48 hours and allowed to germinate, they form a good source of vitamin C.

Deficiency Symptoms

A deficiency of vitamin C results in soft gums, skin haemorrhages, capillary weakness, deterioration in collagen, anaemia, and slow healing of sores and wounds. It may lead to premature ageing, thyroid insufficiency, and lowered resistance to all infections. Its deficiency enhances the toxic effect of drugs and environmental poisons. Mild deficiencies of vitamin C may appear in the form of lassitude, fatigue, anorexia, muscular pain, and greater susceptibility to infection. A prolonged deficiency may cause scurvy.

Healing and Therapeutic Properties

Deficiency of vitamin C can be prevented by eating plenty of fresh citrus fruits like limes, lemons, and oranges. The cheapest sources of vitamin C in India are Indian gooseberries, germinated cereals, grains and pulses, drumstick leaves, and coriander leaves. In case of insufficient intake of vitamin C-rich foods, the

Rich Sources of Vitamin C*

Cereals, Pulses & Legumes	mcg
Red gram, tender	25,000
Peas	9,000
Maize, tender	6,000
Bengal gram, whole	3,000

Vegetables	
Parsley	2,81,000
Drumstick leaves	2,20,000
Turnip greens	1,80,000
Cabbage	1,24,000
Drumsticks	1,20,000
Bitter gourd	88,000
Radish leaves	81,000
Carrot leaves	79,000
Brussels sprouts	72,000
Beet greens	70,000
Celery leaves	62,000
Cauliflower	56,000
Fenugreek leaves	52,000
Cluster beans	49,000
Turnips	43,000
Bathua leaves	35,000
Tomatoes, green	31,000
Spinach	28,000
French beans	24,000
Sweet potatoes	24,000
Round gourds, tender	18,000
Potatoes	17,000
Ladies' fingers	13,000
Brinjals	12,000
Papayas, green	12,000
Lettuce	10,000

Nuts	mcg
Coconut, dry	7,000
Coconut milk	3,000

Fruits	
Indian gooseberries	6,00,000
Guavas, country	2,12,000
Orange juice	64,000
Limes	63,000
Papayas, ripe	57,000
Strawberries	52,000
Limes, sweet	50,000
Lemons, sweet	45,000
Lemons	39,000
Pineapples	39,000
Custard apples	37,000
Lychees	31,000
Oranges	30,000
Raspberries	30,000
Melons, musk	26,000
Mangoes, ripe	16,000
Pomegranates	16,000

Fish & Meat	
Koi	32,000
Indian shard	24,000
Rohu	22,000
Liver, sheep	20,000
Tengra, fresh	18,000

Milk & Milk Products	
Khoa, wholemilk, cow's	6,000
Skimmed milk powder, cow's milk	5,000
Wholemilk powder, cow's milk	4,000

* Values per 100 g edible portions.

deficiency can be overcome by taking 50-100 mg of vitamin C as a daily supplement.

Vitamin C is used therapeutically in huge doses from 100 to 10,000 mg a day. In acute poisoning or infections, 1,000 to 2,000 mg, preferably in injection form, can be administered every one and a half or two hours.

Common Cold. According to Dr Linus Pauling, a Nobel Prize-winning scientist, the regular use of vitamin C in the optimum daily amount will prevent a common cold and if a cold has already appeared, large doses of this vitamin will relieve the symptoms and shorten its duration. However some studies testing supplementation have reported only small moderating effects on the severity and duration of colds.

Infections. Vitamin C is highly acclaimed as a vital factor for the defence of the infected organism. The examination of the urine, blood, or cerebrospinal fluid of patients suffering from an infectious disease will show an abnormally low level of vitamin C. Additional supplies of this vitamin administered to such patients will be retained in the body and not eliminated in the urine. The administration of high doses of vitamin C is thus indicated in an acute state of all infectious diseases. The treatment should be continued and doses gradually decreased until complete recovery.

Stress. The need for vitamin C is so greatly increased during stress that a deficiency can be produced in hours even though the vitamin intake may be as per the recommended daily allowance. The blood vessels become fragile when vitamin C is lacking. Too little of this vitamin can, therefore, lead to a minor injury, such as a small ulcer, and ultimately, result in a major haemorrhage. In tests conducted, it was found that monkeys and guinea pigs lacking in vitamin C developed ulcers. There was no other cause of stress. Guinea pigs put to stress by having one leg immobilised by a splint, developed haemorrhaging ulcers. This was prevented in similarly treated animals by giving them many times the normal requirement of vitamin C.

Atherosclerosis. Experiments have shown that monkeys undersupplied with vitamin C produced cholesterol six times more rapidly than those who received the recommended daily allowance. Administration of upto 50 times of the normal requirement of vitamin C corrected severe atherosclerosis in rabbits and guinea pigs, and resulted in the increased formation of bile acids and the excretion of cholesterol. Administration of large doses of this vitamin to patients suffering from atheros-clerosis and high blood pressure can, therefore, result in a marked decline in their blood cholesterol and a gradual drop in their blood pressure.

Cancer. Any cancer results in severe stress, and this tremendously increases the need for vitamin C. Most cancer patients, especially children with leukemia, show symptoms of bruising, bleeding gums, and often — outright haemorrhaging, characteristic of a vitamin C deficiency. Administration of 4,000 to 6,000 mg of vitamin C daily to patients with inoperable malignancies, inhibits cancer growth and, in some cases, even results in its regression.

Nephritis. A person suffering from any kidney disease can also suffer from a vitamin C deficiency due to stress, medication, and high urinary loss. The danger of haemorrhaging is greatly increased. Even a mild lack of vitamin C can cause blood to appear in the urine. In patients suffering from severe nephritis, administration of large amounts of vitamin C, ranging from 100 mg to 10,000 mg per day, can sometimes quickly stop the passing of bloody urine or haemorrhaging. The intake should be decided upon under medical advice.

Other Diseases. Vitamin C has been used therapeutically in the treatment of several other diseases and conditions like haematemesis(vomiting of blood), nose-bleeding, bleeding piles, melanea(black stools caused by blood in the intestines), erythema nodosum(red nodules in the skin), deep corneal ulcers, anoxia(loss of smell), defective formation of dentine and enamel, dental caries, periodontitis(bleeding from the gums), inflammation of the tongue, delayed growth and development, and rickets. It has been found that adequate intake of vitamin C, along with vitamin B complex, during the entire period of pregnancy, prevents congenital deformities in babies.

Precautions. There are no proven toxic effects of vitamin C, though excessive intake may cause some unpleasant side-effects such as occasional diarrhoea, excess urination, kidney stones, and skin rashes. The dosage should be reduced if any of these symptoms occur.

The 'Sunshine' Vitamin

Vitamin D is commonly known as 'the sunshine vitamin'. It is the most essential vitamin for preventing rickets, which is a known deficiency disease affecting children, and is characterised by defective bone

Recommended Daily Allowance		
Men	.01	mg
Women	.01	mg
Children	.01	mg

formation, disturbance of calcium utilisation in the body, and resulting weakness.

In the 19th century, cod-liver oil was accepted by physicians in Holland, France, and Germany as a therapeutic agent for rickets. Through his classical studies on puppies, E. Mellanby(1918) clearly showed that rickets was a nutritional disease responding to a fat-soluble vitamin present in cod-liver oil.

Research on the chemical nature of vitamin D was initiated in 1924, when H. Steenbock and A. F. Hess demonstrated independently that antiricketic activity could be induced in foods containing certain fat-soluble substances by exposure to ultraviolet light. This discovery of the activation of fat-like substances by ultraviolet rays led to the manufacture of a concentrated vitamin D preparation such as viosterol, long before the pure crystalline vitamin D(calciferol) was isolated in 1935.

Although about ten compounds with vitamin D activity have been identified, the two most important are vitamin D_2 or ergocalciferol, and vitamin D_3 or cholecalciferol.

Vitamin D_3 was found to be identical to the natural vitamin D occurring in fish-liver oils. Vitamin D in foods and in food concentrates is not easily destroyed by heating. It is soluble in fat and fat-solvents and insoluble in water.

While bile is essential for the absorption of vitamin D, fat helps in its absorption too. This vitamin is absorbed from the jejunum of the small intestine and is transported, like vitamin A, in the lymph chylomicrons to the bloodstream. Reserves of the vitamin are found in the liver, skin, brain, and bones, where it is stored for future use. Excretion of vitamin D and its metabolites occurs primarily in the faeces with the aid of bile salts. Very little vitamin D appears in the urine.

Functions in the Body

Vitamin D assists in the assimilation of calcium, phosphorus and other minerals in the digestive tract. It is necessary for the healthy functioning of the parathyroid glands, which regulate the calcium level in the blood. It is very important during infancy and adolescence for the proper formation of teeth and bones. It plays an important role in the prevention of dental caries. Vitamin D protects children against rickets. A good supply of this vitamin during pregnancy benefits the mother and helps to ensure the satisfactory future development of the child.

Sources

Vitamin D is produced from a substance present beneath the skin when sunlight falls upon the surface of the body. This vitamin is not present in any significant degree in foods. Its natural distribution is limited to small amounts in fish oils, *ghee,* eggs, and butter. Compared with fish-liver oil, which is the best source of vitamin D, other foods are quite low in vitamin D.

Rich Sources of Vitamin D*

Fish & Poultry	mcg	Fats & Edible Oils	mcg
Cod-liver oil	175	*Ghee*	2.5
Shark-liver oil	50	Butter	1.0
Halibut-liver oil	5-100		
Eggs	1.5		

* Values per 100 g edible portions.
Note: Sunlight is the most important source of this vitamin.

Deficiency Symptoms

Prolonged deficiency of vitamin D may cause rickets, a disease affecting the whole body. Its most characteristic symptom is the failure of the bones to calcify properly. The growth and maintenance of the normal bones largely depends on this. Lack of vitamin D may lead to tooth decay, pyorrhoea, brittle or soft bones, retarded growth, and poor bone formation in children. It may cause muscular weakness, lack of vigour, deficient assimilation of minerals, and premature ageing. Lack of this vitamin in children can also give rise to improper activity of the parathyroid gland, and result in convulsions.

Healing and Therapeutic Properties

Therapeutically if upto 100 to 125 mcg of vitamin D are taken daily by adults, and half this quantity is taken by children, this is a safe dose. However it should not be taken for longer than one month.

Rickets. Vitamin D plays a very important role in the prevention and treatment of rickets. The therapeutic dose varies from 25 to 125 mcg per day, depending on the severity of the disease. Many preparations under different trade names are available as capsules or palatable syrups, which contain standard amounts of vitamin A and D. For severe cases needing upto 125 mcg per day, a synthetic preparation called calciferol is useful.

Arthritis. Vitamin D is considered extremely beneficial in the treatment of arthritis. It needs to be taken with calcium for the body to be able to utilise it efficiently.

Tooth Decay. Vitamin D has been found beneficial in the treatment of tooth decay. Mellanby proved the importance of this vitamin for tooth nutrition in children. She found that she could control and predict the process of tooth formation in children by the quantum of their vitamin D intake. In certain instances, when generous amounts of vitamin D were given to a child, tooth destruction actually ceased, and the other teeth became harder and firmer.

Bone Repair. Any excess of calcium stored in the long bones serves as a reserve for bone repair when needed. Vitamin D also contributes substantially towards bone repair by increasing calcium absorption through the intestinal wall and reabsorption from the kidney tubules. This vitamin also regulates the deposition of minerals in bones and teeth.

Precautions. Dosages of over 125 mcg taken daily may adversely affect some individuals. Signs of toxicity are unusual thirst, sore eyes, itching on the skin, vomiting, diarrhoea, and an urgent and frequent need to urinate. Abnormal calcium deposits may also be found in the blood-vessel walls, liver, lungs, kidneys, and stomach.

The Anti-Ageing Factor

In 1923 Herbert Evans and Katherine Bishop in California, USA, discovered that there existed a dietary factor which was essential for reproduction in rats. It was given the name vitamin E or anti–sterility factor by Dr E. V. Shute

Recommended Daily Allowance		
Men	15	mg
Women	12	mg
Children	8.3	mg
Infants	4-5	mg

in 1924. It was, however, only in 1936 that Evans and his colleagues finally isolated pure vitamin E from wheat–germ oil. They called it tocopherol. This word is derived from *tocos* meaning child birth, and *pheros* meaning to bear.

Eight different tocopherol compounds with vitamin E activity have been identified uptil now. All of them have the same physiological properties. The tocopherols are yellow, oily liquids, freely soluble in fat solvents. They are not easily destroyed by heat even at room temperature above 100°C or 212° F. Substances which interfere with or destroy vitamin E in the body are iron compounds, synthetic oestrogen, and chlorine or chlorinated water.

Approximately 50 to 85 per cent of vitamin E in the diet is absorbed from the gastro–intestinal tract by a mechanism similar to that of other fat–soluble vitamins. It enters the bloodstream via the lymph. The vitamin is stored in all the tissues, and the tissue stores can provide protection against the deficiency of this vitamin for long periods. About one–third of the vitamin is excreted in the bile and the balance is excreted in the urine.

Functions in the Body

The main functions of vitamin E are to help protect the functioning of cells and the intracellular processes. Vitamin E oxygenates the tissues and reduces the need for oxygen intake markedly. It is essential for normal reproductory functions, fertility, and physical vigour. It prevents unsaturated fatty acids, sex hormones, and fat–soluble vitamins from being destroyed in the body by oxygen.

Vitamin E dilates the capillaries and enables the blood to flow freely into blood-deficient muscle tissue, thus strengthening both the tissues and the nerves supplying them. It dissolves blood clots and also prevents their formation. It does not, however, interfere with the normal clotting of blood. It prevents the formation of excessive scar tissues and in some instances, even melts away unwanted scar tissue. It also promotes urine secretion. Vitamin E is said to be essential for prevention of heart disease, asthma, arthritis, and many other conditions.

Sources

The richest sources of vitamin E are cold–pressed crude vegetable oils, especially wheat germ, sunflower seeds, safflower, and soya bean oils. Eggs, butter, raw or sprouted seeds, and grains — especially whole wheat — are moderately good sources. Meats, fruits, and green leafy vegetables provide small quantities of this vitamin.

Deficiency Symptoms

Deficiency of vitamin E may lead to degenerative changes in the blood capillaries which, in turn, can lead to heart and lung disease, pulmonary embolism, and a brain stroke. Deficiency of this vitamin may also lead to loss of sexual potency. A prolonged deficiency may lead to reproductive disorders, abortions, miscarriages, male or female sterility, as well as muscular disorders.

Healing and Therapeutic Properties

Vitamin E can be used in therapeutic doses from 200 to 2,400 mg daily, depending on the need. It has proved beneficial in the treatment of several disorders. The more important of these disorders are mentioned below.

Sterility. Vitamin E has been used successfully in the treatment of sterility. About 100 mg of this vitamin is given daily in these cases. This vitamin has proved helpful in the prevention of sterility in male animals in laboratory tests. Sterile female animals have also been able to conceive after the administration of large doses of vitamin E.

Abortion and Congenital Anomalies. Vitamin E is used in the prevention of habitual abortion, a tendency towards premature delivery, and congenital irregularities. Research has confirmed that congenital anomalies result from placental inadequacy. Vitamin E has proved to be effective in overcoming this inadequacy. When a woman who has given birth to anomalous infants earlier, discovers that she is pregnant again, she should be given vitamin E, along with a diet rich in protein, calcium, and iron during the entire period of pregnancy. This is an effective protection against infant mortality and infant anomalies.

Administration of vitamin E to males increases the number of spermatozoa which has probably fallen in count due to malnutrition, a sedentary lifestyle, stress, and excessive use of tobacco. In all such cases 100 mg of vitamin E taken daily for at least three weeks, before intercourse, can prevent congenital anomalies.

Dysmenorrhoea. Vitamin E has proved to be beneficial in the treatment of dysmenorrhoea or painful menses. Administration of 200 mg of this vitamin daily during the menstrual period is found to be very effective in this regard.

Menopause. Menopause or the cessation of the menstrual cycle due to ageing, is a critical period in a woman's life. She often undergoes severe tension and several other psychological problems. Vitamin E therapy in doses of 200 mg daily for a month or so will give her great relief from hot flushes, mental tension, sleeplessness, and other symptoms.

Old Age. Vitamin E contributes towards a healthy old age. During this period, one usually feels weak and tired due to bio-chemical changes in the tissues. However regular intake of 200–400 mg of vitamin E a day makes one feel strong and fresh.

Heart Disease. Intake of adequate amounts of vitamin E strengthens the walls of the blood vessels and decreases clotting of blood inside their walls. In a study, 100 patients with heart disease were given 200 mg of vitamin E daily. They were compared with an equal number of patients who were not given this vitamin. The latter experienced four times the number of heart attacks caused by clots. Similarly, 457 patients had no clots while taking vitamin E as compared to 23 clots suffered by 246 patients who were not given the vitamin.

Vitamin E is said to markedly reduce the need for oxygen and is, hence, of particular value for all persons with heart disease. In coronary artery disease, for instance, oxygen starvation is a major problem. Moreover, many deaths from a heart attack are due to oxygen deprivation. When adequate vitamin E(as prescribed) is given, much less of the heart tissue is destroyed, and a patient may survive an attack which otherwise might have proved fatal.

Varicose Veins. A lack of vitamin E is a cause of frequent blood clots which, in turn, play a role in the production of varicose veins. Tests have proved that blood clots which blocked circulation were produced in animals whose diet lacked in vitamin E. When this vitamin was added, formation of these clots stopped. The veins became dilated, and extra blood vessels developed around the areas of the clots quickly. Similarly, giving vitamin E to human beings has been found to prevent clots, and clot formation recurs if vitamin E is discontinued. Varicose veins appear most frequently during pregnancy.

Precautions. Vitamin E is essentially non-toxic, and there are no known toxic effects seen even after the administration of single doses.

Prevents Haemorrhages

Vitamin K is a fat–soluble vitamin. It is essential for the production of a type of protein called prothrombin and other factors involved in the blood–clotting

Recommended Daily Allowance	
Men	70-140 mcg
Women	70-140 mcg
Children	35-75 mcg

mechanism. Hence it is known as an anti–haemorrhagic vitamin.

This vitamin was discovered in 1935 by Dam, who recognised a severe deficiency disease in newly–hatched chicks who were fed on a ration adequate in protein, minerals, and all the known vitamins. The haemorrhages were apparently due to a fall in prothrombin, the clotting agent in the blood. The normal clotting time was restored by administering hog–liver fat or by feeding alfalfa. Dam called the anti–haemorrhagic factor found in these materials vitamin K.

With the help of the Swiss chemist Karrer and his colleagues, H. Dam finally isolated the vitamin in 1939. In the same year, and only a few months later, the successful synthesis of vitamin K was achieved by three different laboratories in USA.

Vitamin K exists in nature in two forms. Vitamin K_1, originally isolated from lucerne(alfalfa), is the only form that occurs in plants. It is a yellow oil, soluble in fat solvents, but only slightly soluble in water. Vitamin K_2 has been found to be produced by many bacteria.

Vitamin K is not easily destroyed by light, heat, or exposure to air. It is, however, destroyed by strong acids, alkalis, and oxidising agents. X–rays and radiation, frozen foods, aspirin, air pollution, and mineral oil are other factors that can destroy vitamin K.

Studies of the liver stores of vitamin K indicate that approximately 50 per cent of the vitamin comes from the diet and 50 per cent from bacterial production in the intestines. Vitamin K is absorbed along with fat in the diet. Bile is essential for its absorption. The absorbed vitamin passes through the lymphatic system to the general circulation. The liver stores appreciable amounts of this vitamin. There is hardly any excretion of vitamin K by the body. Early studies, however, indicate that the major route of excretion of the intravenously administered radioactive vitamin is the faeces.

Functions in the Body

Vitamin K is essential for the prevention of internal bleeding and haemorrhages. It aids in reducing excessive menstrual flow in women. This vitamin is important for the normal functioning of the liver. It is also involved in the energy-producing activities of the tissues, particularly, those of the nervous system.

Sources

Vitamin K is fairly widely distributed in foods. It appears abundantly in cauliflower, cabbage, spinach, alfalfa, yoghurt, soya beans, and, to a lesser extent, in wheat and oats. Animal products contain only a little vitamin K. Cow's milk is a better source than human milk. Vitamin K is also manufactured by bacteria in healthy intestines.

Rich Sources of Vitamin K*

Vegetables	mcg		mcg
Kale	730	Cabbage	130
Turnip greens	650	Lettuce	130
Spinach	420	Asparagus	60
Broccoli	200	Watercress	60

* Values per 100 g edible portions.

Deficiency Symptoms

Primary deficiency of vitamin K in adults has not yet been clearly demonstrated, either by observation of malnourished patients or by dietetic experiments on volunteers. Hence it may be assumed that even the worst diets contain enough of this vitamin to meet normal human needs. A deficiency state would more likely be caused by a failure to absorb or utilise the vitamin. Low vitamin K intake, plus antibiotic therapy, which reduces its production by bacteria, may result in lowered levels of vitamin K in the body.

A deficiency of vitamin K which results in the blood taking longer to clot, may cause severe haemorrhages anywhere in the body. Nosebleeds and bleeding can prove to be life threatening.

Healing and Therapeutic Properties

The discovery and identification, the isolation and synthesis of compounds with vitamin K activity have made the extensive clinical use of this vitamin for the control and the prevention of haemorrhages due to vitamin K deficiency, possible.

Haemorrhages in Newborns. Infants present a special situation in terms of vitamin K because of a limited placental transfer of the vitamin, and because the gut of the newborn is sterile and cannot synthesise the vitamin. Thus some infants require extra administration of vitamin K to prevent haemorrhages. This may be given in a water–soluble or fat–soluble form. If mothers have received any anticoagulant therapy, their infants should be given 2 to 4 mg of vitamin K immediately after birth.

Biliary Obstruction. Vitamin K preparations are invaluable in cases where its absorption has been impaired by lack of bile salts, pancreatic secretions, or other causes of digestive failure. It is an essential pre-operative measure if surgery is contemplated in such cases. This vitamin should be given intramuscularly for three days in a dose of 10 to 20 mg daily, prior to the operation.

Precautions. Vitamin K can be toxic if given in large doses over a prolonged period of time. Symptoms of vitamin K toxicity reported by A. M. Smith and R. P. Custer are diminution of prothrombine in the blood, small haemorrhages, and kidney disorders. In premature infants, there can be jaundice and anaemia.

Airola Paavo. *How to Get Well*. Arizona: Health Plus Pub., 1974.

Aman. *Medicinal Secrets of Your Food*. Mysore: Indo-American Hospital, N. R. Mohalla, 1985.

Clark, Linda. *A Handbook of Natural Remedies for Common Ailments*. New York: Pocket Books, 1977.

Davis, Adelle. *Let's Get Well*. USA: New American Lib., 1972.

Hauser, Gayelord. *The New Diet Does it*. New York: Berkley Publishing Corporation, 1972.

Kordel, Lelord. *Health the Easy Way*. Reprint. New York: Award Books, 1976.

Machlin, Laurence J. *Handbook of Vitamins*. New York: Marcel Dekker, 1984.

Mindel, Earl. *The Vitamin Bible*. First reprint. New Delhi: Allied Publishers Pvt. Ltd., 1983.

Angustine, Jorg, Barbara P. Klein, Deborah A. Becker, Paul B. Venugopal. *Methods of Vitamin Assay*. New York: John Willey and Sons, 1985.

Braunwald, Eugene, Kurt J. Isselbacher, Robert G. Petersdorf, Jean D. Wilson, Joseph B. Martin, and Anthony S. Fauci. *Harrison's Principles of Internal Medicine*. 11th ed. New York: McGraw Hill Book Company, 1988.

Davidson, Stanley, R. Passmore, J. F. Brock, A.S. Truswell. *Human Nutrition & Dietetics*. 6th ed. Great Britain: The English Language Book Society and Churchill Livingstone, 1975.

Mitchell, Rynbergen, Anderson, and Dibble. *Nutrition in Health & Diseases*. 16th ed. Philadelphia: J. B. Lippincott Co., 1976.

Rao, B.S. Narasinga, Y.G. Deosthale, K.C. Pant. *Nutritive Value of Indian Foods*. Revised reprint. Hyderabad, India: National Institute of Nutrition, ICMR, 1993.

PART II
Minerals Your Body Needs

The Chinese do not draw
any distinction between
food and medicine.

—Lin Yutang

Minerals are inorganic substances like sodium, potassium, chlorine, calcium, phosphorus, magnesium, iodine, iron, cobalt, and copper. They are classified into two categories: major and minor, based on the intake level. If more than 100 mg of a mineral is required per day, the mineral is classified as a major mineral. Major minerals include calcium, phosphorus, potassium, sodium, chlorine, magnesium, and sulphur. Minor or trace minerals include boron, chromium, cobalt, fluorine, iodine, iron, manganese, molybdenum, selenium, silicon, vanadium, and zinc.

Plants incorporate minerals from the soil into their own tissues. For this reason fruits, vegetables, grains, legumes, nuts and seeds are often excellent sources of minerals. Minerals — as they occur in the earth in their natural form — are inorganic or lifeless. In plants, however, most minerals are combined with organic molecules. This usually results in better mineral absorption. Green leafy vegetables are the best source of many minerals.

Minerals are vital for good health. Like vitamins they are essential for regulating and building the cells which make up the body. Body cells receive the essential food elements through the bloodstream. They must, therefore, be properly nourished with an adequate supply of all the essential minerals for the efficient functioning of the body.

Minerals help to maintain the volume of water necessary for the life processes in the body. They help draw chemical substances into and out of the cells, and keep the blood and tissue fluids from becoming either too acidic or too alkaline. The importance of minerals, like vitamins, is illustrated by the fact that there are over 50,000 enzymes in the body which direct growth and energy, and each enzyme has minerals and vitamins associated with it. Each of the essential food minerals does a specific job in the body, while some of them do extra work in teams to keep the body cells healthy.

Minerals thus play an important role in bodily functions and are present in every human cell. Although the amount needed may be small, even the lack of the required trace of the mineral is bound to lead to a dysfunction at some level in the body. Less obvious deficiencies may surface as fatigue, irritability, loss of memory, nervousness, depression, and weakness.

The total content of some of the important minerals required in the human body is represented in the diagram on the opposite page.

These inorganic minerals are essential for the proper growth and assimilation of the organic substances, and development of every part of the body.

The body can tolerate a deficiency of vitamins for a relatively long period, but even slight changes in the concentration of the important minerals in the blood may rapidly endanger life.

The role of the more important of these minerals in the body, their deficiency symptoms, and their therapeutic uses are described in the subsequent chapters.

Total Mineral Content Required in the Body

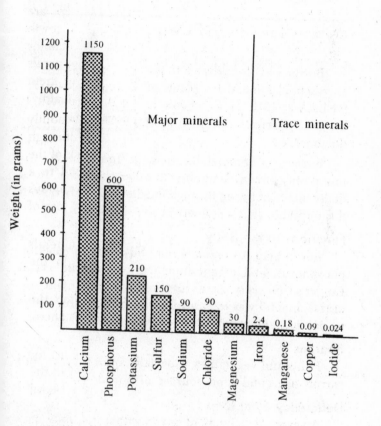

Prevents Tumours and Cysts

Boron was considered to be an essential mineral for plants as far back as 1910. Its exact role in human nutrition is not well documented.

Recommended Daily Allowance
2 mg – adequate in average diet

Boron is a non-metallic element. In the body, it is found only in combination with other chemicals. Most of the intake of boron through the diet is absorbed from the intestine. It is excreted in the urine.

Functions in the Body

Boron helps to regulate the body's use of calcium, phosphorus, and magnesium. During experiments at Rutger's University, it was discovered that the main task of this mineral was to control cell growth. It thus helps to prevent abnormalities in growth.

Sources

Fruits and vegetables, especially apples, pears, and carrots are good food sources of boron.

Deficiency Symptoms

A severe deficiency of boron within the body may be partially responsible for tumours, cysts, and other abnormal growths.

Precautions. A daily intake of over 100 mg of boron can produce toxic symptoms. Boric acid was formerly used as a food preservative, but has been declared unsafe as a food additive by the FAO/WHO Expert Committee.

For Strong Bones

The human body requires more calcium than any other mineral. The body of the infant at birth contains about 27.5 g of calcium, while the adult human body contains about 1,000 to 1,200 g. At least 99 per cent of this quantity is found in the bones and teeth, giving them strength and rigidity.

Recommended Daily Allowance		
Men	400	mg
Women	400	mg
Preg. Wo.	1000	mg
Lact. Wo.	1000	mg
Children	600	mg
Infants	500	mg

The remaining one per cent, which is in the blood, muscles, and nerves, plays an important role in regulating important physiological functions.

Calcium is a white, malleable, metallic element. Among other substances it is found in chalk, gypsum, and limestone. In the body it is found in various combinations such as calcium carbonate, calcium phosphate, calcium fluoride, and calcium sulphate. All these compounds are formed from the calcium carbonate in the organism. Large quantities of fat, oxalic acid, and phytic acid in the food can prevent proper calcium absorption.

Not all the calcium that is present in foods is available to the body. The absorption and retention of this mineral depends on its intake as well as other factors. Normally, approximately 20 to 40 per cent of this mineral is absorbed from the intestinal tract into the bloodstream. The amounts absorbed, however, may be greatly increased during periods of rapid growth when mineral needs are high. Absorption of calcium also depends on the healthy condition of the stomach and intestines and adequate supply of vitamins B_{12}, D, C, and phosphorus.

Calcium is excreted mostly through the urine and the stools. Excretion in the stools is increased when there is deficiency of fats in the food and when there is defective absorption of calcium in the intestine. It is estimated that the daily excretion of calcium through the urine varies between 100–300 mg in men and 100–250 mg in women. This quantity, however, varies and the excretion becomes less during calcium deficiency.

Functions in the Body

Calcium plays an important role in the maintenance of health. It has been called the prime instigator of vital activity. This mineral is essential for the proper development of bones and teeth. It is necessary for the normal action of the heart and all muscle activity. It aids the clotting process of the blood and stimulates enzymes in the digestive process.

Calcium is required for proper foetal growth, for normal health of the mother during pregnancy and lactation, and for the secretion of breast milk. It speeds all healing processes and controls the conduction mechanism in the nerve tissues so that messages travel fast enough for the functioning of the body. It is essential for proper utilisation of phosphorus and vitamins D, A, and C.

Sources

Milk and milk products are the most important sources of calcium in readily available form. One litre of cow's milk contains 0.12 per cent of calcium. Green vegetables such as cassia, amaranth, turnip greens, cauliflower, carrots, and leaves of colocasia, drumsticks, fenugreek, and radishes are excellent sources of calcium. Other good sources are mustard seeds, dried coconut, and almonds. Finger millet(*ragi*) is the cheapest natural source of calcium, containing about 0.3 to 0.36 per cent. Fish too is a rich source of calcium.

Deficiency Symptoms

Deficiency of calcium causes changes in the bones and muscles. Calcium-deficient people look pale and listless, get tired, and become lazy. They are more sensitive to cold weather. They become nervous and suffer from mental derangements. Sweating around the head even during cold weather is the most obvious symptom of calcium deficiency in all ages. Deficiency of calcium may cause porous and fragile bones, tooth decay, heart palpitations, muscle cramps, insomnia, and irritability.

Children who are born to calcium-deficient mothers generally suffer from calcium deficiency. In such children calcium deficiency becomes more prominent if there is no adequate supply of calcium, proteins, minerals, and vitamins in the form of whole milk, fresh fruits, and vegetables. These children fail to grow or develop healthy and strong bones. They lack appetite and if fed forcibly, may bring out all the food and milk. They suffer from indigestion and diarrhoea. They suffer from late and defective teething, and are prone to having emaciated necks and enlarged heads. Deficiency of calcium lowers the body resistance and these children become an easy prey to respiratory and intestinal infections.

Deficiency of calcium in young girls causes late puberty, irregular menstruation, excessive bleeding with crampy pain, anaemia, and lowered state of body resistance against infections. In case of an inadequate supply of calcium during pregnancy, the development of the foetus continues by drawing the reserve calcium from

Rich Sources of Calcium*

Cereals	mg
Finger millet	344
Rice, bran	67
Wheat flour, whole	48
Bajra	42
Wheat, whole	41
Wheat germ	40

Pulses & Legumes

Kidney beans	260
Soya beans	240
Bengal gram, whole	202
Moth beans	202
Split black gram	154
Green gram, whole	124
Split kesari	90
Peas, roasted	81
Cowpeas	77
Split green gram	75
Peas, dry	75
Split red gram	73

Vegetables

Fetid cassia, dried	3,200
Colocasia leaves, dried	1,546
Curry leaves	830
Amaranth, spinosus	800
Turnip greens	710
Cauliflower greens	626
Amaranth, paniculates	530
Fetid cassia, fresh	520
Colocasia leaves, black variety	460
Drumstick leaves	440
Lotus stems, dry	405
Amaranth, gangeticus, tender	397
Fenugreek leaves	395
Pumpkin leaves	392
Parsley	390
Beet greens	380
Carrot leaves	340
Radish leaves	265
Tamarind leaves, tender	101

Nuts & Oilseeds

	mg
Mustard seeds	490
Coconut, dry	400
Almonds	230
Groundnut cake	213
Pistachio nuts	140
Walnuts	100
Water melon seeds, kernal	100
Chilgozas	91
Groundnuts	90
Cashew nuts	50

Fruits

Banyan tree figs	364
Currants, black	130
Dates, dried	120
Apricots, dry	110
Limes	90
Raisins	87
Bael fruit	85
Lemons	70
Mulberries	70
Indian gooseberries	50
Guavas, hill	50

Fish, Meat & Poultry

Mutijella, dried	7,240
Bhagon, dried	6,235
Shrimp, small, dried	4,384
Chingri, goda, dried	3,847
Chela, dried	3,590

	mg		mg
Chingri, small, dried	3,539	*Khoa*, skimmed milk, buffalo's	990
Parsey, dried	2,231	*Khoa*, wholemilk, cow's	956
Mango fish, dried	1,597		
Bombay duck, dried	1,389	Wholemilk powder, cow's milk	950
Bhetki, dried	939	Cheese	790
Rohu	650		
Katla	530	*Khoa*, wholemilk, buffalo's	650
Cat fish	230	Cottage cheese, buffalo's milk	480
Mutton, muscle	150		
Beef meal	68	Milk, buffalo's	210
Eggs	60	Cottage cheese, cow's milk	208
Milk & Milk Products			
Skimmed milk powder, cow's milk	1,370	Curd, cow's milk	149
		Milk, cow's	120

* Values per 100 g edible portions.

---

the bones, but the mother usually suffers from a difficult labour. Bleeding, lack of breast milk, poor concentration of the mind, a prolonged lying-in period — these are all common due to calcium deficiency after childbirth.

Healing and Therapeutic Properties

A large increase in the dietary supply of calcium is needed in tetany(a condition marked by abnormal excitability of the nerves and muscles), and when the bones are decalcified due to poor calcium absorption, as happens in tetany, rickets, and osteomalacia. A liberal quantity of calcium is also necessary when excessive calcium has been lost from the body, as in hyperparathyroidism(over-action of the parathyroid gland) or chronic kidney disease. In such cases, plenty of milk should be given. If this is insufficient, calcium lactate should be given. A teaspoon of calcium lactate weighs about two grams and provides 400 mg of absorbable calcium. An effective therapeutic dose is three teaspoons, given three times a day in water before meals. It provides about 3.6 g of calcium.

Insomnia. Insomnia can frequently be dispelled by increased intake of calcium, because it causes the nerves and muscles to relax. Those who do not sleep well are advised to take three calcium tablets with a glass of warm milk on retiring. This is said to bring a sound, refreshing sleep.

Menopause. Calcium has been found useful in menopausal disorders. During menopause, a lack of ovarian hormones can result in a severe calcium deficiency. A larger than usual intake of calcium may therefore help greatly. Hot flushes, night sweats, leg cramps, irritability, nervousness, and mental depression associated with this condition can be overcome by giving liberal quantities of this mineral.

Cramps and General Irritability. Relatively quick results from intake of calcium in therapeutic doses (between 600 and 1,200 mg) have been reported in conditions involving irritability of the nerves and muscles such as in menstrual cramps, leg cramps, and general irritability. In these cases, calcium seems to do its work by swiftly moving into the bloodstream and soft tissues of the body.

Arthritis. Studies have shown that arthritis can be relieved by a liberal intake of calcium. Several patients suffering from this disease discovered that their joint pains were either relieved or stopped completely after taking this mineral in therapeutic doses. This treatment should be continued for at least four months to achieve beneficial results.

Precautions. Excessive daily intake of calcium of over 2,000 mg may lead to hypercalcaemia.

The Natural Disinfectant

Chlorine exists in the form of a salt(chloride) in the human body. It is present mostly in the extracellular fluid.

Recommended Daily Allowance		
Men	300-900	mg
Women	300-900	mg
Children	160-500	mg

Chlorine is a greenish-yellow, poisonous, gaseous element with a suffocating odour. In the body it is mostly present as sodium chloride or common salt, which performs various essential functions.

Functions in the Body

Chloride is essential for the proper distribution of carbon dioxide and the maintenance of osmotic pressure in the tissues. It is necessary for the manufacture of glandular hormone secretions. It prevents the building of excessive fat and autointoxication. Chloride regulates the alkali-acid balance in the blood. It works with potassium in a compound form. Potassium chloride is also essential for the production of hydrochloric acid in the stomach, which is needed for proper protein digestion. It is involved in the maintenance of proper fluid and electrolyte balance in the system.

Sources

Chloride is found in barley, wheat, and other grains and pulses, green leafy vegetables, and fruits like melon, and pineapple.

Rich Sources of Chlorine*

Cereals, Pulses & Legumes	mg		mg
		Drumstick leaves	423
Barley	91	Curry leaves	198
Peas, roasted	73	Fenugreek leaves	165
Peas, dry	59	Tamarind leaves,	
Bengal gram, whole	58	tender	94
Wheat, whole	47	Amaranth, gangeticus	88
Jowar	44	Colocasia leaves	72
Bajra	39	Spinach	54
Split Bengal gram	39	Brinjals	52
Maize, dry	33	Cauliflower	34
Red gram, tender	22	**Fruits**	
Split green gram	25	Melons, musk	80
Vegetables		Melons, water	21
Lotus stems, dry	444		

* Values per 100 g edible portions.

The chloride that we take is mostly in the combined form of sodium chloride. Hence the foods that contain large quantities of sodium also contain chloride in the same proportion and vice versa.

Deficiency Symptoms

Deficiency of chloride can occur when sodium chloride is restricted during the active phase of general oedema or hypertension. The symptoms produced are the same as those which occur with sodium chloride deficiency. Excessive loss of salt from the body due to perspiration can result in heat cramps. Deficiency may lead to loss of hair and teeth. It may also result in impaired digestion of foods and derangement of fluid levels in the body.

Healing and Therapeutic Properties

Chlorine is widely used in disinfecting water for drinking. It is also used in swimming pools. Taken in the form of eusol which contains hypochlorus acid, chlorine is used to disinfect chronic ulcers, but this usage is limited because its action is stopped by the presence of excessive organic matter.

Salt intake during summer should be sufficient to meet the body's requirements as there is excessive vomitting and diarrhoea due to heat.

Precautions. The fumes of chlorine are poisonous. After a patient has apparently recovered from exposure to chlorine gas, he may develop lung oedema and become seriously ill. In such a case the appropriate treatment is administration of oxygen. Chlorine is used for bleaching, and some household bleaches which contain hypochlorites give off chlorine to produce their effect. It they are swallowed, the stomach, gullet, and mouth can be seriously irritated.

Promotes Glucose Tolerance

Chromium is present in traces in all organic matter and seems to be an essential mineral. Chromium levels are higher in infants than in adults. The total body content of chromium in adults is 5 to 10

Recommended Daily Allowance	
Men	50-200 mcg
Women	50-200 mcg
Children	20-200 mcg
Infants	10-60 mcg

mg. As a person grows older, he is able to retain less chromium in the body. The concentration in human tissues varies greatly in different parts of the world, depending on dietary habits and on the amount of chromium in water supplies.

Chromium is a greyish-white metallic element. Little is known about the chemical forms in which it occurs in individual foods.

Most of the intake of chromium is not absorbed and urinary excretion is low.

Functions in the Body

Chromium plays an important role in the metabolism of carbohydrates and fats. It works with insulin in the metabolism of sugar. It seems to increase the effectiveness of insulin, thereby facilitating the transport of glucose into the cells and not allowing the blood glucose levels to rise. It helps to take protein where it is needed and also aids in growth.

Sources

The main food sources of chromium are betel leaves, arecanut, and nuts.

Rich Sources of Chromium*

Cereals	mcg		mcg
Italian millet	30	Onion stalks	39
Finger millet	28	Carrots	17
Bajra	23	Beet root	12
Barley	16	Colocasia leaves	11
Wheat, whole	12	Drumstick leaves	10
Pulses & Legumes		**Nuts & Oilseeds**	
Bengal gram, whole	32	Arecanuts, raw	473
Peas, dry	32	Arecanuts, processed	386
Kidney beans	29	Cashew nuts	163
Soya beans, black	29	Almonds	161
Soya beans, white	28	Walnuts	101
Lentil, whole	24	Mustard seeds	63
Split black gram	12	Groundnuts	48
Black gram, whole	12	**Fruits**	
Red gram, whole	10	Custard apples	26
Vegetables		Pomegranates	22
Betel leaves	137	Tomatoes, ripe	15
Mangoes, green	50	Jack fruit, ripe	13
Bottle gourd	46	Pineapples	11

* Values per 100 g edible portions.

Deficiency Symptoms

A deficiency of chromium can cause impairment of glucose tolerance, which can lead to diabetes. It is also a suspected factor in arteriosclerosis. In some areas, protein-energy malnutrition appears to be associated with chromium deficiency.

Healing and Therapeutic Properties

Chromium has been found beneficial in the prevention and treatment of high blood pressure. It also works as a preventive against diabetes. Studies have also found that chromium supplements control total cholesterol and triglyceride levels, and raise the HDL(the good cholesterol). In some patients with impaired glucose tolerance, especially children with protein malnutrition, the tolerance to glucose has shown improvement after the patients have been given chromium supplements. It is also claimed that a chromium supplement can control the symptoms of epilepsy.

Precautions. Excessive intake of this mineral, however, can lead to occupational dermatitis(eczema) and lung cancer.

Converts Iron into Haemoglobin

The first conclusive evidence to show that copper was an essential element for the formation of haemoglobin in rats suffering from iron-deficiency anaemia, emerged from the studies of E. B. Hart and his co-workers in 1928.

Recommended Daily Allowance	
Men	2 mg
Women	2 mg
Children	.05-0.1 mg*

There is approximately 75 to 150 mg of copper in the adult human body. Newborn infants have higher concentrations of copper than adults. The liver, brain, kidneys, heart, and hair contain relatively high concentrations. The average serum copper levels are higher in adult females than in males. The serum copper levels also increase significantly in women during pregnancy and when taking oral contraceptives.

In the human body, copper is a constituent of several enzymes and is found in combination with several proteins in the blood.

Ceruloplasmin, a copper-containing plasma enzyme, catalyses the oxidation of the ferrous ion to ferric ion, and thereby enables iron to be trapped by transferrin (a protein transporting iron in the blood). It is then transported to tissues for the synthesis of iron-containing compounds, especially haemoglobin.

Copper is mostly absorbed at the level of the duodenum in the intestine. Approximately 32 per cent

* Value per kg of body weight.

of the copper in the diet is absorbed. Excess copper is excreted in the bile.

Functions in the Body

Copper helps the conversion of iron into haemoglobin. It stimulates the growth of red blood cells. It is also an integral part of certain digestive enzymes. It makes the amino acid — tyrosine — usable, enabling it to work as the pigmenting factor for the hair and skin. It is also essential for the utilisation of vitamin C.

Sources

Molluscs and shellfish are rich sources of copper, as are betel leaves, arecanuts and other nuts. Soft water contains more copper than hard water and water from the tap contains more copper than reservoir water. However, the latter is a better source of copper than water taken directly from the stream.

Deficiency Symptoms

Copper deficiency may result in weakness of the body, digestive disturbances, and impaired respiration. Anaemia due to copper deficiency has not been reported in adults. All medicinal iron preparations contain traces of copper. Infants, especially those who are born premature, may develop copper deficiency, which usually presents itself as chronic diarrhoea, and later develops into anaemia which does not respond to iron. Copper deficiency has been reported in protein energy malnutrition.

Healing and Therapeutic Properties

Menke's Syndrome. This is a rare, genetically determined failure of copper absorption. This condition leads to progressive mental retardation, failure to keratinise hair which becomes kinky, hypothermia, low concentrations

Rich Sources of Copper*

Cereals	mg	Nuts & Oilseeds	mg
Italian millet	1.40	Arecanuts, processed	2.54
Barley	1.19	Walnuts	1.67
Bajra	1.06	Cashew nuts	1.66
Wheat, whole	0.68	Coconut, dry	1.00
Wheat flour, whole	0.51	Almonds	0.97
Finger millet	0.47	Groundnuts	0.90
Rice flakes	0.37	Mustard seeds	0.83

Pulses & Legumes		Fruits	
Lentil, whole	1.87	Oranges	0.58
Kidney beans	1.45	Custard apples	0.43
Soya beans, black	1.38	Pears	0.40
Lentil	1.37	Pomegranates	0.34
Split Bengal gram	1.34	Lychees	0.30
Peas, roasted	1.32	Bael fruit	0.21
Peas, dry	1.29	Grapes, pale green	
Red gram, whole	1.23	variety	0.20
Split red gram	1.20	Papayas, ripe	0.20
Bengal gram,		Tomatoes, ripe	0.19
whole	1.18	Limes, sweet	0.17
Black gram, whole	1.05	Bananas, ripe	0.16
		Guavas, country	0.14
Vegetables		Pineapples	0.13
Betel leaves	2.32	Plums	0.13
Lotus stems, dry	1.22		
Radishes, white	0.40	Fish	
Celery leaves	0.30	*Chingri, goda,* dried	1.40
Beetroot	0.29	Mango fish, dried	1.20
Tomatoes, green	0.19	*Tapra,* dried	0.71
Colocasia leaves	0.18	Chela, dried	0.51
Onions, big	0.18	*Bata,* small varieties	0.17
Potatoes	0.16	*Chitai*	0.17
Cauliflower	0.13	*Koi*	0.16
Brinjals	0.12	Singhi	0.15
Round gourds, tender	0.12	Indian shard	0.14
Fenugreek leaves	0.10	Parsey, fresh	0.14

* Values per 100 g edible portions.

of copper in the plasma and liver, and degenerative changes in the body.

Arthritis. Copper is believed to be beneficial in the treatment of arthritis, as this mineral helps to strengthen the muscular system. Drinking water kept overnight in a copper container is said to relieve this disease, as this water has traces of copper. For the same reason, wearing a copper ring or bracelet may also help. People in ancient times, including Egyptians, Scandinavians, South American and North American Indians, wore copper bracelets for the relief of aches and pains. In Peru, the Incas wear copper even today and the natives claim that they have no rheumatic troubles.

Precautions. Taking copper in excess is poisonous and food cooked in copper vessels with poor tin-plating can cause severe vomiting and diarrhoea with abdominal pain. Drinking acid drinks in copper vessels can also produce the same symptoms.

For Healthy Teeth

In 1805, J. L. Gay-Lussac first detected fluorine in the bodies of animals. Although the recommended daily allowance of fluorine is normally met through drinking water, the importance of this element in nutrition was realised when high incidence of chronic endemic fluorosis in men and farm animals was detected in 1931 in certain parts of India.

There is a strong affinity between calcium and fluorine. These two elements work together, particularly in the outer parts of bones. They are found in the enamel of the teeth and the shiny and highly polished bone surfaces.

Fluorine is pungent and corrosive. It belongs to the same group of elements as chlorine, bromine, and iodine. In the body, it is found in combination with other constituents of the body.

Ingested fluorides are completely ionised and rapidly absorbed, and distributed throughout the extracellular fluid in a manner similar to chloride. However the levels in the blood and tissues are so low that it has been difficult to make any reliable analysis. Fluoride is rapidly excreted in the urine, even by those suffering from severe kidney disease. The relationship of the urinary output of flourine in comparison to the total intake is complicated and related to the state of the bones.

Sources

Fluorine is found in Bengal gram, cereals — especially rice, some leafy vegetables, and most of all in dry tea leaves.

Fluorine is found in small amounts in normal bones and teeth. Since water containing 1 to 2 parts per million(ppm) prevents dental caries and does not do any harm, the fluorine requirements of the body are met by the quantity normally present in drinking water in most regions.

Rich Sources of Fluoride*

Cereals	ppm**		ppm**
Rice	7.7	Potatoes	1.9
Wheat flour, milled	5.4	Capsicums	1.7
Wheat, whole	2.9	French beans	1.5
Bajra	1.9	Tomatoes	1.4
Pulses		Cluster beans	1.2
Bengal gram flour, milled	8.1	**Fruits**	
Split Bengal gram	3.8	Apples	1.7
		Oranges	1.7
Vegetables		Mangoes	1.3
Amaranth, leaves	6.1	Bananas	1.1
Carrots	3.4	**Fish & Poultry**	
Cucumbers	2.5	Prawns	2.7
Onions	2.1	Pomphret, white	2.1
Spinach	2.1	Eggs	1.5
Brinjals	2.0	**Beverages**	
Cabbage	1.9	Tea, dry leaves	56.6

* Values per 100 g edible portions.
** Fluoride content in parts per million.

Deficiency Symptoms

Studies have shown that animals fed on a fluorine-deficient diet develop dental caries. This disease can be prevented by incorporating fluorine at a level of

1 to 2 parts per million(ppm) in the diet. Studies on dental caries in human beings have shown that the incidence in children is high in areas where the drinking water contains less than 0.5 ppm fluorine, and low in areas where the water contains 1 to 2 ppm fluorine. It has further been shown that the addition of 1 ppm fluorine to drinking water significantly reduces the incidence of dental caries.

Healing and Therapeutic Properties

Deficiency of fluorine can be prevented by sufficient intake of fresh vegetables, fish, fruits, tea, and dried meat.

Precautions. Signs and symptoms of dental fluorosis have been observed in several countries where the drinking water contains excessive amounts of fluorine, that is, from 3 to 5 ppm. In these cases, the enamel of the teeth loses its lustre and chalky white patches are found irregularly over the surface of the teeth. In severe cases, there is a marked loss of enamel with the tooth surface acquiring a corroded appearance.

Prolonged drinking of water containing excessive amounts of fluorine over 10 ppm can lead to fluorine intoxication. Workers handling fluoride-containing minerals can also suffer from this problem. This may result in pathological changes in the bones. There may be an increased density and hypercalcification of the bone of the spine, pelvis, and the limbs. The ligaments of the spine may also become calcified, producing a 'poker back'. Neurological disturbances secondary to the changes in the vertebral column are common.

Prevents Goitre

Iodine was one of the first minerals to be recognised as vital for good health. It is still considered one of the most important.

Recommended Daily Allowance		
Men	150	mcg
Women	150	mcg
Children	83	mcg

Goitre has been known since prehistoric times. In the Middle Ages, centuries before iodine itself was discovered, physicians in Europe treated goitre with burnt sponge, a substance rich in iodine. This is a remarkable example of the efficacy of folk medicine and the acumen of early physicians.

In practically all countries, there are areas where iodine is lacking in the soil and water. Only one country — Japan — is virtually free from this disease and this is attributed to the relatively high consumption of seaweed as a foodstuff. Seaweed, according to Mc Clendon, a well-known nutritionist, contains about a thousand times as much iodine as any other food. It has been used in the Japanese diet for many generations without any apparent adverse effects.

Iodine was accidentally discovered in burnt seaweed by B. Courtois in 1811, and first isolated by Fyfe in 1819. In 1896, E. Baumann discovered that the thyroid gland, when compared with the other tissues, was very rich in iodine. In 1917, Drs Marine and O. P. Kimball carried out an extensive survey among American school children and conclusively proved the value of iodine both in preventing and curing simple goitre.

Iodine is greyish-black in colour. When heated, it yields corrosive fumes of a rich violet colour. In the human body, it forms an essential component of thyroxine, the main hormone produced by the thyroid gland. The excessive consumption of certain foods like cabbage, cauliflower, and raddish can cause iodine deficiency. These foods contain a substance which reacts with the iodine present in the food and makes it unsuitable for absorption.

Dietary iodine is absorbed from the gastro-intestinal tract into the blood. The amount of iodine present in the body of an adult is estimated to be about 25 milligrams. Most of it is concentrated in the thyroid gland, where it is stored in the form of thyroglobulin, a complex of protein and iodine. About 30 per cent is removed by the thyroid gland for the synthesis of the thyroid hormone, thyroxine, and the rest is excreted by the kidneys. Proteolytic enzymes(those which split up the proteins during digestion) break down this compound, and thyroxine and a small amount of triiodothyronine are excreted into the circulating blood. When the amount of the thyroid hormone in the serum is decreased, the pituitary gland releases a thyroid-stimulating hormone which causes the thyroid gland to produce more cells and to increase in size in an attempt to manufacture more hormones. This results in enlargement of the thyroid gland, which is also called simple goitre.

Functions in the Body

The chief storehouse of iodine in the body is the thyroid gland. Thyroxine, which is secreted by this gland, contains iodine. This iodine is obtained from the food that is eaten.

Thyroxine, the thyroid hormone, controls the basic metabolism and oxygen consumption of tissues. It controls the utilisation of sugars. It regulates the rate of energy production and body weight and promotes proper growth. It increases the heart rate as well as urinary calcium excretion. It improves mental alacrity and promotes healthy hair, nails, skin, and teeth.

Sources

The best dietary source of iodine is iodised salt. Sea foods and spinach also contain reasonable quantities of iodine.

Rich Sources of Iodine*

	mcg		mcg
Iodized table salt	7,600	Spinach	20
Sea foods	30-300	Eggs	9

* Values per 100 g edible portions.

Deficiency Symptoms

Cretinism occurs in children whose diet lacks iodine. A cretin is a dwarfed child who is mentally retarded, has an enlarged thyroid gland and defective speech, and a gait that is clumsy. His skin is rough, and hair, sparse. Such a child usually has brittle nails, bad teeth, and is prone to anaemia.

Among adults, myxoedema can result from an iodine deficiency, affecting the adequate production of the thyroid hormone. The symptoms of this disease are a slower rate of metabolism, thickening of the skin, loss of hair, and general physical and mental sluggishness. Such persons also have enlarged thyroid glands.

A dietary lack of iodine may lead to anaemia, fatigue, lethargy, loss of interest in sex, a slow pulse, low blood pressure, and a tendency towards obesity.

A serious deficiency may result in high blood cholesterol and heart disease.

Iodine is so important to life that a mere three and a half grains of this precious element stands between intelligence and idiocy! The thyroid gland can manufacture the hormone thyroxin only from organic iodine taken through the mouth.

Healing and Therapeutic Properties

Small doses of iodine are of great value in the prevention of goitre in areas where it is endemic, and are of value in treatment in the early stages. Larger doses have a temporary value in patients with hyperthyroidism who are being prepared for surgical operation.

Precautions. There are no known toxic effects from natural iodine. However, iodine as a drug can be harmful if prescribed incorrectly.

Purifies the Blood

The haemoglobin content of the red blood cells is made up of certain proteins and iron. In a normal healthy adult there is about 15 g of haemoglobin per 100 ml of blood. Each gram of haemoglobin contains about 3.5 mg of iron.

Recommended Daily Allowance	
Men	28 mg
Women	30 mg
Preg. Wo.	38 mg
Children	26-40 mg

The normal body of an adult contains about 4 to 5 g of iron. About 60 to 70 per cent of this iron is present in the haemoglobin. Iron stores in the liver, spleen, and bone marrow account for the next largest concentration of iron — that is, about 30 to 35 per cent. Small amounts of iron are found in the muscles as myoglobin, as also in the blood serum and in every cell as a constituent of certain enzymes. Iron is present in the body in combination with other body constituents.

All healthy persons absorb about 2 to 10 per cent of iron from food, depending on its nature. But in persons who are deficient in iron, the amount absorbed increases upto 50 per cent from ingested foods.

The main sites of absorption are the stomach and the upper part of the small intestine. Absorption of iron is enhanced when there is a deficiency of iron in the body or there is a need for increased blood formation.

Iron is stored in the liver, spleen, and intestinal mucosa. The stores of iron as well as the iron released from the disintegration of red blood cells is available to the body for the synthesis of haemoglobin. Hence the iron in our bodies is used very efficiently, and is not normally used up or destroyed but converted and utilised again and again.

Iron is excreted along with the bile, stools, scaling of the skin, and sweating. It is, therefore, advisable to take an extra quantity of iron-rich foods during summer to compensate the iron loss.

Functions in the Body

Iron is essential for life. It is necessary for the production of haemoglobin. Haemoglobin is composed of four iron-containing heme groups. The heme is responsible for the characteristic colour and the oxygen-carrying capacity of the blood. Iron thus enables the blood to carry oxygen throughout the body and is of great value in helping to remove carbon dioxide from the tissues.

Myoglobin(an oxygen-carrying protein containing iron) in the muscle tissue is related to blood haemoglobin in both structure and function. It supplies oxygen to the muscles and removes carbon dioxide. Iron increases resistance to stress and disease. It aids growth and prevents fatigue.

Sources

The best food sources of iron are wholegrain cereals, pulses and legumes, and fish. The best plant sources are green leafy vegetables such as dry lotus stems, cauliflower greens, and turnip greens; fruits such as black currants, water melons, raisins, and dried dates.

Enzymes and hydrochloric acid in the stomach are needed for proper assimilation of iron. Older people are often anaemic in spite of plenty of iron in their diet

Rich Sources of Iron*

Cereals	mg		mg
Rice bran	35.0	Colocasia leaves,	
Rice flakes	20.0	green variety	10.0
Bajra	8.0	**Nuts & Oilseeds**	
Rice, puffed	6.6	Mustard seeds	7.9
Wheat germ	6.0	Coconut, dry	7.8
Wheat, whole	5.3	Pistachio nuts	7.7
Wheat flour, whole	4.9	Water melon seeds	7.4
Jowar	4.1	Cashew nuts	5.8
Rice, raw, hand-		Almonds	5.1
pounded	3.2	**Fruits**	
Pulses & Legumes		Currants, black	8.5
Soya beans	10.4	Melons, water	7.9
Bengal gram, roasted	9.5	Raisins	7.7
Moth beans	9.5	Dates, dried	7.3
Cowpeas	8.6	Apricots, dry	4.6
Lentil	7.6	Custard apples	4.3
Peas, dry	7.0		
Peas, roasted	6.4	**Fish & Meat**	
Split kesari	6.3	*Chingri, goda*, dried	49.6
Split Bengal gram	5.3	Mango fish, dried	41.2
Kidney beans	5.1	*Chingri*, small, dried	27.9
Bengal gram, whole	4.6	*Tapra,* dried	19.3
Green gram, whole	4.4	Bombay duck, dried	19.1
		Beef meal	18.8
Vegetables		Parsey, dried	17.4
Lotus stems, dry	60.6	Bhetki, dried	15.0
Cauliflower greens	40.0		
Turnip greens	28.4	**Milk & Milk Products**	
Bengal gram leaves	23.8	*Khoa,* wholemilk,	
Cowpea leaves	20.1	buffalo's	5.8
Parsley	17.9	*Khoa,* skimmed milk,	
		buffalo's	2.7

* Values per 100 g edible portions.

because they lack sufficient hydrochloric acid in their stomachs. For these reasons, iron-containing fruits which possess their own enzymes and acids needed for iron digestion and assimilation, are the most reliable sources of dietary iron.

Deficiency Symptoms

Iron deficiency is generally caused by severe blood loss, malnutrition, infections, and by excessive use of drugs and chemicals. Severe blood loss can occur due to a major injury to blood vessels, or rupture of aneurysms, perforation of internal organs, incomplete abortion, and severe menstrual bleeding. Repeated pregnancies, prolonged breast feeding, and excessive sweating during summer also reduce the iron content in the blood. The volume of fluid in the body is also reduced.

Deficiency of iron in the diet may cause nutritional anaemia, lowered resistance to disease, a general rundown condition, pale complexion, shortness of breath on manual exertion, and loss of interest in sex. The patient may suffer from mental depression and irritability.

When there is severe blood loss, the body becomes pale and cold with profuse sweating. The patient becomes extremely exhausted and finds great difficulty in breathing. The mind becomes dull and the patient may become unconscious. If blood transfusion or some other method is not adopted immediately to prevent further blood loss and shock, the patient may die soon.

Healing and Therapeutic Properties

Eating foods rich in iron regularly and keeping the gastro-intestinal tract healthy is one of the safest and more potent methods of preventing iron deficiency.

Different types of anaemias may be due to different causes. However only iron-deficiency anaemia responds to the supplementary intake of iron.

Precautions. Iron stored in the body in excess quantities is harmful.

The Alcoholic's Balm

All human tissues contain small quantities of magnesium. The adult human body contains about 25 g of this mineral, the greater part of which is present in bones in combination with phosphate

Recommended Daily Allowance	
Men	350 mg
Women	300 mg
Children	150-200 mg
Infants	150 mg

and carbonate. Bone ashes contain less than one per cent magnesium.

About one-fifth of the total magnesium in the body is present in the soft tissues inside the cells, where it is mainly bound to protein. The bones seem to provide a reserve supply of this mineral in case of a shortage elsewhere in the body.

Magnesium is a light, silver-white, malleable, and ductile metallic element. It burns with a very hot, bright flame and is used to form light-weight alloys. Biochemists call magnesium the 'cool, alkaline, refreshing, sleep-promoting mineral'. It helps to keep one calm and cool during the sweltering summer months. Intake of diuretics and alcohol can render magnesium ineffective.

Active absorption of this mineral occurs in the ileum of the small intestine. Magnesium may compete with and decrease calcium absorption from the intestine. The parathyroid hormone, parathormone, which controls serum calcium levels, has a similar effect on magnesium. Almost twice the amount of magnesium is stored in bones as compared with soft tissues. Bone magnesium

126

is, however, not readily exchanged with the magnesium of soft tissues.

Since a greater part of magnesium in the diet is not absorbed, it is excreted in the stools. About one-third of the amount ingested is excreted in the urine. Urinary excretion is reduced in magnesium deficiency. The magnesium content in the blood is about 2 to 3 mg/ 100 ml.

Functions in the Body

Magnesium helps to keep the nerves relaxed. It is necessary for all muscular activity. It is an activator of most of the enzyme systems involved in the metabolism of carbohydrate, fat, and protein. It is necessary for the activation of alkaline phosphatase, an enzyme involved in calcium and phosphorus metabolism. Magnesium also helps in the utilisation of vitamins B and E. It functions with other minerals such as calcium, sodium, and potassium in maintaining fluid and electrolyte balance. Adequate levels of magnesium are necessary for normal neuromuscular contractions. This mineral is also involved in the production of lecithin. It prevents the building up of cholesterol and consequent artherosclerosis.

Magnesium promotes a healthier cardiovascular system and thus helps prevent heart attacks. It aids in fighting depression. It helps to prevent calcium deposits in kidneys and gallstones. It also provides relief from indigestion.

Sources

Magnesium is widely distributed in foods. It is a part of the chlorophyll in green vegetables. Other good sources of this mineral are nuts, soya beans, alfalfa, apples, figs, lemons, peaches, almonds, wholegrains, brown rice, sunflower seeds, and sesame seeds. Cereals and vegetables normally contribute more than two-thirds of the daily magnesium intake.

Rich Sources of Magnesium*

	mg		mg
Cereals		Onion stalks	104
Jowar	171	Spinach	64
Rice, parboiled,		Celery leaves	52
hand-pounded	157	Cluster beans	47
Maize, dry	139	Drumstick leaves	42
Bajra	137	Bitter gourd, white	36
Finger millet	137	Colocasia leaves	32
Wheat flour, whole	132	Lettuce	30
Rice flakes	101	Potatoes	30
Rice, parboiled,		**Nuts**	
milled 5%	91	Almonds	373
Italian millet	81	Cashew nuts	349
Pulses & Legumes		Walnuts	302
Soya beans, black	238	**Fruits**	
Moth beans	225	Mangoes, ripe	270
Kidney beans	184	Plums	147
Soya beans, white	175	Custard apples	84
Bengal gram, whole	169	Grapes, pale green	
Black gram, whole	154	variety	82
Split Bengal gram	130	Pomegranates	44
Split black gram	130	Bananas, ripe	41
Peas, roasted	122	Jambu fruit	39
Split red gram	90	Pineapples	33
Lentil	74	Melons, musk	31
Vegetables		Cherries, red	27
Betel leaves	447	Guavas, country	24
Radishes, pink	196	Jack fruit, ripe	24
Lotus stems, dry	168	Peaches	21
Amaranth,			
gangeticus	122		

* Values per 100 g edible portions.

Deficiency Symptoms

Magnesium deficiency is unlikely to arise in human beings due to an inadequate intake of foods containing it. Deficiency may, however, occur under the same metabolic condition that leads to a lack of potassium, namely, excessive loss due to chronic diarrhoea.

Magnesium deficiency has been observed in patients with certain clinical conditions where magnesium intake or absorption has been decreased and magnesium excretion increased. These conditions include chronic alcoholism, diabetes, malabsorption syndrome, renal disease, disorders of the parathyroid gland, and postsurgical stress.

Continuous deficiency of magnesium also causes a loss of calcium and potassium from the body with consequent deficiencies of these minerals. Deficiency can lead to kidney damage and kidney stones, muscle cramps, atherosclerosis, heart attack, epileptic seizures, nervous irritability, marked depression and confusion, impaired protein metabolism, and premature wrinkles. Magnesium deficiency increases an individual's susceptibility to high blood pressure.

Healing and Therapeutic Properties

Alcoholism. Chronic alcoholics often show a low plasma magnesium concentration and a high urinary output. They therefore require extra magnesium intake, especially in an acute attack of delirium tremens.

Kidney Stones. By increasing the solubility of calcium in the urine, magnesium prevents recurrence of kidney stones. Magnesium, together with vitamin B_6 or pyridoxine, has also been found effective in the prevention and treatment of kidney stones.

When needed, magnesium can be taken in a therapeutic dose of upto 700 mg a day. Magnesium chloride is the best form of supplementary magnesium, although other forms can also be used. Magnesium salts taken by mouth are both diuretic and laxative. The cathartic(stool loosening) action is due to the slow absorption of magnesium from the intestine and the consequent drawing of water into the gut.

Heart Attacks. Low levels of magnesium have been found in persons who suddenly die of heart attacks. The magnesium deficiency may lead to a spasm in the coronary arteries, which in turn, reduces the flow of blood and oxygen to the heart. Magnesium therapy offers some protection against heart disease.

Precautions. Large amounts of magnesium over an extended period of time, can be toxic if the calcium and phosphorus intakes are high. Supplements of magnesium should not be taken after meals as the mineral neutralises stomach acidity.

For the Growing Years

The nutritional importance of manganese was discovered in 1936-37, when A. H. Norris and his co-workers and T. P. Lyons and Insko reported the development

Recommended Daily Allowance	
Men	3 mg
Women	3 mg
Children	1.6 mg

of bony malformation in poultry fed on a manganese-free diet. Studies of L. S. Hurley and G. J. Everson and their associates in 1961 threw more light on the relationship of manganese to growth, bone development, reproduction, and the functioning of the central nervous system.

Manganese is found in the body as a trace element and is essential for life. The human body contains 10 to 20 mg of this element which is widely distributed throughout the tissues. It is found in high concentration in the mitochondria of cells.

Manganese is a hard, brittle, greyish-white metallic element. It is readily oxidised and forms an important component of certain alloys. If manganese is breathed in excess, in the form of dust or fumes, it can lead to a condition very much like Parkinson's disease wherein tremors develop in the hands and fingers.

Only three to four per cent of the manganese present in the diet is absorbed from the intestine and reaches the blood. It is stored in the blood and liver. Serum manganese levels are almost always elevated following a myocardial infarction.

Manganese is excreted in the faeces. The urine contains only traces of this element. High calcium intakes have been shown to increase the faecal excretion of manganese.

Functions in the Body

Manganese is an important component of many enzyme systems which are involved in the metabolism of carbohydrates, fats, and proteins. In combination with choline, it helps in the digestion and utilisation of fat. Manganese helps to nourish the nerves and brain and assists in the proper coordinative action between the brain, nerves, and muscles in every part of the body. It is also involved in normal reproduction and the function of mammary glands.

Sources

Nuts, whole grains, and dried legumes are excellent sources of manganese.

Rich Sources of Manganese*

Cereals & Pulses	mg	Vegetables	mg
Finger millet	5.49	Betel leaves	4.47
Green gram, whole	2.47	Onion stalks	0.74
Soya beans, black	2.35	Spinach	0.56
Wheat, whole	2.29	Coriander leaves	0.50
Wheat flour, whole	2.29	Drumstick leaves	0.37
Soya beans, white	2.11	Amaranth, gangeticus	0.36
Kidney beans	1.60	Colocasia	0.28
Bengal gram, whole	1.21	Sweet potatoes	0.22
Bajra	1.15	**Nuts & Oilseeds**	
Rice, parboiled, hand-pounded	1.10	Coconuts, dry	6.24
Split Bengal gram	1.05	Arecanuts, processed	2.83
Lentil, whole	1.04	Walnuts	2.62
Barley	1.03	Mustard seeds	2.56
Split green gram	1.02	Almonds	1.88
Black gram, whole	1.01	Cashew nuts	1.42
		Groundnuts	1.10

* Values per 100 g edible portions.

Deficiency Symptoms

A prolonged deficiency of manganese may cause retarded growth, digestive disorders, abnormal bone development, and deformities. It may also cause male and female sterility and sexual impotence in men. However, the human body obtains sufficient manganese through normal dietary intake, so a deficiency syndrome is rare.

Healing and Therapeutic Properties

Since manganese deficiency rarely occurs, this element is seldom prescribed.

Precautions. Toxic symptoms have been reported to occur in mine workers due to inhalation of dust from manganese ores. The symptoms are blurred speech, tremors of the hands, and a spastic gait.

For General Well-Being

Molybdenum is an essential trace mineral found in animals and human beings. The amount of this mineral present in plants varies greatly, depending on the

Recommended Daily Allowance	
Men	500 mcg
Women	500 mcg
Children	266 mcg

soil. A relatively higher amount is present in plants which are grown on neutral or alkaline soils with a high content of organic matter, and a lower amount in those grown on acid, sandy soils.

Molybdenum is a hard, heavy, and silver-white metallic element of the chromium group. It occurs only in combination with other chemicals in the body.

The excretion of molybdenum in the urine may be upto half the total daily intake.

Functions in the Body

Molybdenum is essential for the synthesis of haemoglobin and absorption of iron. It functions as a component in several enzymes, including those involved in alcohol detoxification, uric acid formation, and sulphur metabolism. This trace mineral aids in carbohydrate and fat metabolism.

Sources

Foods rich in proteins and iron are said to contain molybdenum in sufficient concentration. Whole grains, pulses and legumes, leafy vegetables, and nuts are the main food sources of this element.

Rich Sources of Molybdenum*

Cereals	mcg		mcg
Finger millet	102	Split black gram	425
Rice, parboiled,		Green gram, whole	304
hand-pounded	78	Split red gram	283
Italian millet	70	Red gram, whole	222
Bajra	69	Split Bengal gram	195
Rice, parboiled,		Lentil, whole	171
milled 5%	68	Bengal gram, whole	154
Rice, milled 5%	58	**Vegetables**	
Rice, parboiled,		Coriander leaves	1,120
milled 10%	54	Fenugreek leaves	400
Wheat, whole	51	Amaranth, gangeticus	130
Rice, milled 10%	45	Cabbage	78
Jowar	39	Cucumbers	70
Wheat flour, whole	39	Potatoes	70
Maize, dry	38	Onions	30
Pulses & Legumes		**Nuts & Oilseeds**	
Cowpeas	1,890	Gingelly seeds	204
Black gram, whole	810	Groundnuts	166
Peas, dry	638	Mustard seeds	89
Split green gram	446	Safflower seeds	54

* Values per 100 g edible portions.

Molybdenum, like other trace minerals, is not destroyed by cooking. A varied diet, including foods which are rich in molybdenum, should negate the necessity of taking any supplements, with a few exceptions.

Deficiency Symptoms

It has been seen that animals on a low molybdenum diet do not grow normally, thus inferring that a deficiency of this mineral can be a contributory factor in some disturbances of iron metabolism. A deficiency can also lead to dental caries. It has been reported that the rates of dental caries are lower than average in children brought up in areas where the soil has a high molybdenum content. A molybdenum deficiency has been suggested as a cause for sulphite sensitivities, because sulphite oxidase, the enzyme that detoxifies sulphites, is molybdenum-dependent.

Healing and Therapeutic Properties

Molybdenum is considered beneficial in the prevention of anaemia. It also promotes general well-being.

Precautions. Toxic reactions to molybdenum are not common. However, a very high incidence of gout in some areas of Armenia has been attributed to high intakes of molybdenum from local plants.

The Body Energiser

Phosphorus is a mineral colleague of calcium within the body. Calcium by itself cannot be responsible for good teeth and bones or nourish the brain and nerves. A proper balance of

Recommended Daily Allowance		
Men	800	mg
Women	800	mg
Children	440	mg

phosphorus must be present in the bloodstream for the effective performance of these tasks.

An adult human body contains about 400-700 g of phosphorus as phosphates. At least two-thirds of this amount is found in chemical combination with calcium in the bones and teeth, and the rest in other tissues. Phosphorus is essential for the proper utilisation of not only calcium but also other minerals like iron, magnesium, potassium, and sodium.

The inorganic phosphorus content of blood serum in normal human adults ranges from 2.5 to 4.0 mg/ 100 ml, and in children from 4.0 to 5.0 mg/100ml. In individuals suffering from rickets, the level of phosphorus is reduced to less than 3 mg/100 ml.

Phosphorus is a soft, non-metallic element found in the body only in combination with other substances. As a result, it is neither luminous nor inflammable. In the human body, phosphorus is a part of the ATP (adenosine triphosphate) and ADP(adenosine diphosphate) — the energy transporting systems in the cells, and is also a component of the phospholipids. Too much iron, aluminium, and magnesium can render phosphorus ineffective.

Phosphorus is absorbed in the small intestine as inorganic phosphates. Phosphorus present in an organic combination such as phytic acid, is hydrolysed to inorganic phosphate before absorption. Since the enzyme, phytase, is not present in human digestive juices, phytin phosphorus is absorbed only to a very slight extent in human beings. Phosphorus present in animal foods such as milk, meat, and eggs is absorbed to a greater extent than that present in cereals and legumes, as the latter exists mostly in the form of phytic acid.

The kidneys are the major pathway of excretion of the absorbed phosphorus. The retention of phosphorus in children on different diets has been reported to vary from 10 to 40 per cent. The retention of phosphorus depends on various factors like the quantity of phosphorus ingested, the calcium content of the diet, the form in which phosphorus exists in the diet, and vitamin D intake.

Functions in the Body

Phosphorus is indispensable for all active tissues. In combination with calcium, it feeds the nerves. It aids the growth of hair and helps counteract fatigue. This mineral is important for the regular functioning of the heart and for normal kidney functioning.

Phosphorus is essential in the chemical processes involved in the utilisation of carbohydrates and fats. It liberates their energy at the rate demanded by the body. It also helps in regulating the acid-alkaline balance of the blood, which is vital for the maintenance of health and prevention of disease.

Phosphorus is also necessary for the formation of the phospholipids — lecithin and cephalin — which are

Rich Sources of Phosphorus*

Cereals

	mg
Rice bran	1,410
Wheat germ	846
Wheat flour, whole	355
Maize, dry	348
Wheat, whole	306
Bajra	296
Italian millet	290
Finger millet	283
Rice, parboiled, hand-pounded	280

Pulses, Legumes & Vegetables

	mg
Soya beans	690
Carrots	530
Kidney beans	410
Split green gram	405
Split black gram	385
Peas, roasted	345
Bengal gram, roasted	340
Split Bengal gram	331
Green gram, whole	326
Bengal gram, whole	312
Split red gram	304
Peas, dry	298
Lentil	293
Moth beans	230

Nuts & Oilseeds

	mg
Water melon seeds, kernal	937
Mustard seeds	700
Chilgozas	494
Almonds	490
Cashew nuts	450
Pistachio nuts	430
Walnuts	380
Groundnuts, roasted	370

Fish

	mg
Chela, dried	2,342
Shrimp, small, dried	1,160
Chingri, goda, dried	828
Silver belly	741
Singhi	650
Mango fish, dried	595
Bhola	580
Seer	572
Tapra, dried	552
Sole, malabar	524
Mushi, dried	507
Boal	490
Folui	450
Tengra, dried	400

Meat

	mg
Liver, sheep	380
Beef meal	324

Milk & Milk Products

	mg
Skimmed milk powder, cow's milk	1,000
Wholemilk powder, cow's milk	730
Khoa, buffalo's milk, skimmed	650
Khoa, wholemilk, cow's	613
Cheese	520
Khoa, wholemilk, buffalo's	420

* Values per 100 g edible portions.

integral parts of a cell structure and also act as intermediates in fat transport and metabolism. This mineral is also an essential constituent of the nucleic acid and nucleo-proteins of body cells.

Sources

The most important food sources of phosphorus are wholegrain cereals, milk, and fish. Vegetables such as carrots, and leafy vegetables; fruits like black currants, raspberries, raisins, and apricots are fairly good sources. Other sources of this mineral are soya beans, lentils, and other pulses and legumes.

Deficiency Symptoms

A phosphorus deficiency may cause loss of weight, retarded growth, reduced sexual powers, and general weakness. It may result in poor mineralisation of the bones, and a deficient nerve and brain function. Conditions associated with calcium deficiency may also occur due to phosphorus deficiency. Deficiencies of phosphorus are however rare, as it is one of the elements available in large quantities in most diets.

Healing and Therapeutic Properties

While taking calcium in therapeutic doses to make up for calcium deficiency conditions or for treating certain ailments, it is advisable to take that calcium supplement in which phosphorus has been added in the correct proportions. This is necessary as calcium cannot achieve its objectives unless phosphorus is present in the required proportion.

Precautions. There are no known toxic effects of phosphorus.

To Prevent Acidosis

Potassium, one of the most important minerals, is essential for the very life of every cell. It is also among the most generously and widely distributed of all the tissue minerals.

Recommended Daily Allowance		
Men	1.7-5.5	g
Women	1.7-5.5	g
Children	0.9-3	g

Potassium is found principally in the intracellular fluid. A small amount of potassium in the extracellular fluid is necessary for normal muscular activity.

The average adult human body contains 120 g of potassium and 245 g of potassium chloride. Out of this body potassium, 117 g is found in the cells and 3 g in the extracellular compartment. Formation of sulphate and phosphate of potassium also takes place from the food potassium in the body.

Potassium is a bluish-white metallic element. It is highly reactive and never found free in nature. It plays an important role as a catalyst in energy production and in the synthesis of glycogen and protein. Liberal use of alcohol, coffee, sugar, and diuretics can lead to depletion of potassium.

Potassium absorption occurs mainly in the small intestine. In healthy people on a normal diet, about 90 per cent of potassium is excreted in the urine. Increased amounts of potassium are found in the urine whenever the tissues are losing potassium. Perhaps the most important cause is a breakdown of cellular proteins such as occurs in diabetes, under-feeding, and after an injury. Any condition giving rise to acidosis is liable to cause cellular depletion of potassium. In patients given diuretics to increase the output of sodium and water in the urine, an important side-effect is an increase in potassium excretion.

In a healthy person the faeces contain very small amounts of potassium. The digestive juices contain large amounts but this is normally reabsorbed in the gut. However, diarrhoea may cause large losses in the stool. Loss of potassium from the skin is usually negligible.

Functions in the Body

Potassium is important as an alkalising agent. It maintains a proper acid-alkaline balance in the blood and tissues. It prevents hyperacidity. This mineral is essential for muscle contraction and is, therefore, important for the proper functioning of the heart, especially for maintaining a normal heartbeat. It promotes the secretion of hormones and helps the kidneys in detoxification of blood. Potassium prevents female hormonal disorders by stimulating the hormone production. It is involved in the proper functioning of the nervous system and helps to overcome fatigue. It also assists in reducing blood pressure.

Sources

Potassium is widely distributed in foods. Pulses such as green gram, cow peas, red gram, and black gram; and vegetables like lotus stems and sword beans are rich in potassium. Other good sources are legumes, leafy vegetables, and fruits such as bael, sweet limes, peaches, and apricots.

Rich Sources of Potassium*

Cereals	mg	Fruits	mg
Finger millet	408	Bael fruit	600
Bajra	307	Limes, sweet	490
Wheat flour, whole	315	Peaches	453
Maize, dry	286	Apricots, fresh	430
Wheat, whole	284	Loquats	390
Italian millet	250	Melons, musk	341
Rice flakes	154	Cherries, red	320
		Lemons	270
Pulses & Legumes		Plums	247
Split green gram	1,150	Indian gooseberries	225
Cowpeas	1,131	Mangoes, ripe	205
Split red gram	1,104		
Moth beans	1,096	**Fish, Sea Food & Meat**	
Split black gram	800	Rohu	288
Peas, roasted	750	Mutton, muscle	270
Split Bengal gram	720	Prawns	262
Lentil, whole	629	Singhi	223
		Beef muscle	214
Vegetables		*Koi*	195
Lotus stems, dry	3,007	Indian shard	183
Sword beans	1,800	Bhetki	173
Colocasia	550	Liver, goat	160
Brussels sprouts	477	Katla	151
Sweet potatoes	393	*Magur*	147
Amaranth,		*Chitai*	119
gangeticus	341		
Drumstick leaves	259	**Milk & Milk Products**	
Potatoes	247	Milk, cow's	140
Papayas, green	216	Curd, cow's milk	130
Spinach	206		
Brinjals	200		
Bitter gourd, green	171		
Tomatoes, green	114		

* Values per 100 g edible portions.

Deficiency Symptoms

Potassium deficiency is most unlikely in healthy individuals because normal food supplies sufficient quantities of this mineral. However potassium deficiency may occur during gastro-intestinal disturbances accompanied by severe vomiting and diarrhoea, diabetic acidosis, potassium-losing nephritis, and potassium loss during steroid therapy and that of similar drugs. Both mental and physical stress can also lead to potassium deficiency.

Potassium deficiency causes undue body tiredness, palpitations of the heart, cloudiness of the mind, nervous shaking and excessive perspiration of the hands and feet, and great sensitivity of the nerves to cold. It may also result in slow healing of ulcers and fractures.

Healing and Therapeutic Properties

Whenever possible, potassium deficiency should be corrected by increased dietary intake or supplementation with potassium salts. Potassium chloride is the salt of choice. It may be given in the form of an elixir or as tablets.

Low Blood Sugar. The use of potassium has been found beneficial in the treatment of low blood sugar — a condition characterised by lassitude, fatigue, apathy, tension, nervousness, weakness, trembling, sweating, and headaches. These symptoms usually start in the morning and continue throughout the day, if one has not eaten well the night before. An intake of sugar and potassium chloride brings almost immediate relief.

Muscle Abnormalities. Potassium is valuable for muscle abnormalities. In a study, healthy volunteers given refined foods deficient in potassium, for a week, developed muscle weakness, extreme fatigue, constipation, and mental apathy. All these symptoms disappeared immediately when 10 g of potassium chloride was given to them. Studies have also shown that severe potassium deficiency can result in muscles becoming weak, lax, soft, or partially paralyzed. Recovery, however, takes place within a short time after taking potassium in large doses.

Sciatica. Increasing potassium intake can often help to alleviate discomfort from leg cramps and sciatica. This is due to the role of potassium in nerve function. Large quantities of vegetable juices, along with increased potassium supplements, can tackle this problem successfully.

Precautions. The toxic effect of potassium is manifested in the muscles and the heart. Muscular weakness and mental apathy are generally marked. High concentration of potassium in the blood is found only in association with other severe diseases such as renal failure and adrenal insufficiency. In these conditions the potassium can leak out into the blood from the damaged cells.

A Special Friend to Women

Selenium acts as a micronutrient or trace element in the human body. Its distribution in the earth's crust varies from place to place. Its content of water varies even more greatly. The amount present in foods also varies widely. Males appear to have a greater need for

Recommended Daily Allowance	
Men	40-70 mcg
Women	45-65 mcg
Preg. Wo.	75 mcg
Lact. Wo.	75 mcg
Children	20-30 mcg
Infants	10-15 mcg

this mineral. About half the supply of their bodies is concentrated in the testicles and parts of the seminal ducts adjacent to the prostrate gland.

Selenium is a grey, crystalline element of the sulphur group. It is an antioxidant and its biological activity is closely related to vitamin E. It is excreted in the semen.

Functions in the Body

Selenium acts with vitamin E as a non-specific antioxidant to protect cell membranes and tissues. Both of them prevent or slow down the ageing process and hardening of tissues. Selenium aids in maintaining youthful elasticity in tissues.

Sources

Wholegrain cereals like wheat germ, barley, and wholewheat bread are the best sources of selenium.

Deficiency Symptoms

Low levels of selenium put people at higher risk of cancer, cardiovascular disease, inflammatory diseases,

Rich Sources of Selenium*

Cereals	mcg	Vegetables & Fruits	mcg
Wheat germ	111	Turnips	27
Barley	66	Garlic	25
Wholewheat bread	66	Orange juice	19
Bran	63		
Oats	56		
Brown rice	39		

* Values per 100 g edible portions.

and other conditions associated with increased free-radical damage, including premature ageing and cataract formation.

Healing and Therapeutic Properties

Selenium has been found beneficial in the prevention and treatment of Keshan disease. This is a syndrome endemic to the Keshan province in China where the soil is deficient in selenium. Keshan disease is characterised by degeneration of the muscle fibres of the heart. During their child-bearing years, women are particularly susceptible to this disease. Selenium binds cadmium and other metals and mitigates their toxic effects.

This mineral also helps in the regeneration of the liver after damage, especially by cirrhosis. It is useful in alleviating hot flushes and menopausal distress. It helps in the prevention and treatment of dandruff. It is believed to neutralise certain carcinogens and provide protection from some types of cancer.

Precautions. Selenium toxicity occurs in animals, but human beings who have consumed vegetables grown in soil containing high selenium content, show no ill effects. Selenium poisoning has been reported due to ingestion of water containing large amounts of the metal. In rare cases, it can result in patchy baldness(alopecia), abnormal nails, emotional instability, and lassitude.

The 'Beauty' Mineral

Silicon is an essential trace mineral. Only minute amounts of this element are present in the tissues and the actual amount required by the body has not been determined so far.

Silicon is a widely distributed non-metallic element. It is second only to oxygen in abundance in the biosphere. Pure silicon is found in the form of white crystals in matured bamboo stems. This mineral and its salts are poorly soluble in water.

Functions in the Body

Silicon is essential for the proper functioning of nerve cells and tissues, and the synthesis of vitamin B_1 or thiamine in the human body. It controls the transmission of nerve impulses. It contributes greatly to the strength and integrity of bones everywhere in the body. It is also essential for the growth of hair, nails, and teeth, and is, therefore, often called the 'beauty mineral'. It makes the eyes bright and protects the skin from becoming flabby. It is beneficial in all healing processes and protects the body against many diseases, such as tuberculosis, irritations in the mucous membranes, and skin disorders.

Sources

The main food sources of silicon are apples, oranges, cherries, raisins, almonds, peanuts, raw cabbage, onions, endives, carrots, eggplants, pumpkin, red beets, celery, cucumber, fish, honey, and corn. An increased need for silicon is best met by increasing the consumption of whole grains, because they are rich sources of absorbable silicon.

Deficiency Symptoms

Deficiency of silicon in animals causes retarded growth and abnormal bone development. A deficiency in human beings can lead to soft brittle nails, ageing symptoms of the skin such as wrinkles, thinning or loss of hair, poor bone development, osteoporosis(a condition of brittle bones caused by hormonal changes or lack of calcium or vitamin D). The chief symptom of silicon deficiency is sensitiveness to cold: one always feels cold even in the hot months.

Precautions. Toxicity of silicon can lead to chronic fibrosis of the lungs. Its reckless use can cause irreparable damage. This mineral should therefore be administered only on the advice of a physician.

Indispensible for Life

Man has been consuming sodium chloride(the chemical name for common salt) from as far back as history has been recorded. The body of a healthy person weighing about 65 kg contains 256 g of

Recommended Daily Allowance	
Men	10-15 g
Women	10-15 g
Children	5-10 g

sodium chloride. Of this, just over half is found in the extracellular fluid. About 96 g is found in the bones and less than 32 g in the cells.

Sodium is a silver-white, highly reactive, alkaline, metallic element. It is soft and malleable. It is normally found inside the body and outside it in combination with other elements. It is essential for life and is present in the fluids of the body outside the cells. It is usually taken in the form of sodium chloride.

Sodium is almost completely absorbed from the gastro-intestinal tract in the normal individual, but substantial losses may occur due to vomiting and diarrhoea. Most of the sodium consumed is excreted by the kidneys, with variable amounts being lost through the skin and stools. The sodium balance in the body is controlled by the hormone aldosterone, which is secreted by the adrenal gland. When the need for sodium increases, increased amounts of aldosterone are secreted which increase the reabsorption of sodium ions by the kidney tubules.

Skin losses may increase greatly when there is profuse perspiration due to strenuous physical exertion in a hot environment. Under such circumstances, salt depletion may be accompanied by heat exhaustion. Salt tablets may be taken with a liberal amount of water in this condition.

Functions in the Body

Sodium is the most abundant cation in the extracellular fluid of the body. It acts with other electrolytes, especially potassium, in the intracellular fluid, to regulate the osmotic pressure and maintain proper water balance within the body. It is a major factor in maintaining the acid-base equilibrium, in transmitting nerve impulses, and in relaxing muscles. It is also required for glucose absorption and for the transportation of other nutrients across cell membranes.

Sources

Vegetables like dry lotus stems and leafy vegetables are rich in sodium, as are a variety of pulses and legumes. Fruits, fish, and meat also contain a substantial amount of sodium.

Deficiency Symptoms

Deficiency of sodium is caused by excessive sweating, prolonged use of diuretics, or chronic diarrhoea. Deficiency may lead to nausea, muscular weakness, heat exhaustion, and mental apathy.

Healing and Therapeutic Properties

In case of mild deficiency of sodium chloride, taking a teaspoon of common salt in a pint of water or in any fruit juice, quickly restores health. In severe conditions, however, administration of sodium chloride in the form of normal saline by an intravenous route may be resorted to.

Precautions. The adverse effects of excessive sodium chloride in the body can be rectified by avoiding the

Rich Sources of Sodium*

Cereals	mg		mg
Maize, tender	51.7	Tomatoes, green	45.8
Wheat flour, whole	20.0	Mangoes, green	43.0
Wheat, whole	17.1	Celery leaves	35.5
Maize, dry	15.9	Round gourd, tender	35.0
Finger millet	11.0	**Fruits**	
Rice flakes	10.9	Lychees	124.9
Bajra	10.9	Melons, musk	104.6
Jowar	7.3	Bananas, ripe	36.6
Pulses & Legumes		Pineapples	34.7
Red gram, tender	93.0	Apples	28.0
Bengal gram, whole	73.2	Melons, water	27.3
Lentil, whole	40.1	Mangoes, ripe	26.0
Split black gram	39.8	**Fish & Meat**	
Moth beans	29.5	Rohu	101.0
Split red gram	28.5	Bhetki	66.0
Green gram, whole	28.0	*Koi*	64.0
Split green gram	27.2	*Magur*	58.0
Vegetables		Singhi	53.0
Lotus stems, dry	438.0	Beef muscle	52.0
Amaranth,		Indian shard	52.0
gangeticus	230.0	Katla	50.0
Fenugreek leaves	76.1	*Chitai*	34.0
Radishes, pink	63.5	Mutton, muscle	33.0
Spinach	58.5	**Milk & Milk Products**	
Lettuce	58.0	Milk, cow's	73.0
Cauliflower	53.0	Curd, cow's milk	32.0
		Milk, buffalo's	19.0

* Values per 100 g edible portions.

Note: Sodium present in foods is not adequate to meet the daily
requirement. Hence sodium chloride(salt) has to be included
in the diet.

---

use of common salt. Foods rich in salt such as salted
nuts, biscuits, meat, fish, chicken, eggs, cheese, dried
fruits, spinach, carrots, and radishes should be avoided.
However, low sodium foods like cereals, sugar, honey,

fresh fruits, brinjals, cabbage, cauliflower, tomatoes, potatoes, onions, peas, and pumpkin can be eaten.

Oversupply of sodium is a more common problem because of overuse of dietary sodium chloride or common salt. Too much sodium may lead to water retention, high blood pressure, and even stomach ulcers.

The point then is that getting used to a decreased amount of salt in the diet, is a matter of habit. What is salty to one person may be bland to another. Fortunately, getting used to less salt in the food does not take long.

For Glowing Hair and Skin

The greater part of the sulphur present in the human body is contained in the two sulphur-containing amino acids, methionine and cysteine.

Recommended Daily Allowance
Provided sufficiently in high-protein diet

Sulphur is a pale yellow, non-metallic element. In the body sulphur is found only in combination with some other constituents of the body. It does not exist in a free state.

Sulphur from foods is absorbed as an organic compound and after metabolism, it is converted into sulphate and excreted in the urine.

Functions in the Body

Sulphur is essential for the synthesis of vitamin B_1. It helps in the digestion of fats and controls the metabolism of carbohydrates. It is essential for healthy hair, skin, and nails. Along with B complex vitamins, it aids the liver in bile secretion.

It is believed that sulphur ejects some of the waste and poisonous matter from the system. It helps to keep the skin clear of blemishes and makes it glossy.

Sources

The main sulphur-containing foods are red gram, green gram, and leafy vegetables. A diet sufficient in protein is generally considered to be adequate in sulphur.

Rich Sources of Sulphur*

Cereals	mg		mg
Finger millet	160	Celery leaves	102
Bajra	147	Brinjals	44
Barley	130	Potatoes	37
Wheat flour, whole	122	**Fruits**	
Maize, dry	114	Jackfruit, ripe	69
Rice flakes	105	Melons, water	42
Pulses & Legumes		Plums	33
Red gram, tender	494	Melons, musk	32
Split green gram	214	Peaches	26
Peas, dry	189	Pineapples	20
Moth beans	180	Lychees	19
Split red gram	177	Mangoes, ripe	17
Split black gram	174	Guavas, country	14
Split Bengal gram	160	Pears	14
Vegetables		Papayas, ripe	13
Lotus stems, dry	258	Pomegranates	12
Cauliflower	231	Tomatoes, ripe	11
Brussels sprouts	212	Apples	7
Fenugreek leaves	167	Bananas, ripe	7
Drumstick leaves	137		

* Values per 100 g edible portions.

Deficiency Symptoms

Deficiency of sulphur may interfere with the healthy growth of hair and nails.

Healing and Therapeutic Properties

Sulphur creams and ointments have been remarkably successful in treating a variety of skin problems.

Precautions. There are no known toxic effects of sulphur.

Good for the Heart

Vanadium is a rare, silver-white metallic element. It is present in the human body in minute quantities. During recent research on laboratory animals, it has been identified as an essential element. The implications of these findings in human nutrition are not fully known.

Recommended Daily Allowance	
Men	1-4 mcg
Women	1-4 mcg

Functions in the Body

Vanadium helps in the metabolism of cholesterol and sugar in the body, thereby preventing the occurrence of heart attacks.

Rich Sources of Vanadium*

Cereals	mcg		mcg
Corn	15	Radishes	5
Buckwheat	10	Onions	5
Wheat, whole	5	Beets	4
Oats	3	Lettuce	2
Millet	2	**Nuts & Oilseeds**	
Vegetables		Peanut oil	11
Green beans	14	Sunflower seed oil	4
Cabbage	10	Olive oil	3
Carrots	10	Sunflower seeds	3
Garlic	10	**Fruits**	
Parsley	8	Apples	3
Tomatoes	6	Plums	2

* Values per 100 g edible portions.

Deficiency Symptoms

There is no evidence to show that man suffers from either deficiency or excess of dietary vanadium.

Healing and Therapeutic Properties

On the basis of experiments conducted on animals, conflicting claims have been made that this trace mineral can prevent or promote dental caries.

Precautions. Vanadium can prove to be toxic if taken in synthetic form.

Hastens Healing

The human need for zinc is small, but its role in growth and well-being is enormous, starting even before birth. The entire body of a normal man weighing 70 kg may contain 1.4 to 2.3 g of zinc. Zinc is present in small amounts

Recommended Daily Allowance	
Men	10-15 mg
Women	10-15 mg
Children	10 mg
Infants	3 mg

in all tissues. The bones, teeth, and the pancreas contain slightly higher amounts of zinc than other tissues. Whole blood contains about 0.7 mg/100 ml, while blood serum or plasma contains 0.1 mg/100 ml.

The importance that zinc played towards the growth and well-being of the albino rat was demonstrated by W. R. Todd in 1934. This was confirmed by other research workers on mice and birds. In 1939, Keilin and J. I. Mann showed that zinc was a constituent of the enzyme carbonic anhydrase. Zinc has also been found in some other enzymes, such as in the pancreatic hormone insulin.

Zinc is a bluish-white, metallic element. It is present in the body mostly in combination with other constituents of the body.

About 20 to 30 per cent of the zinc in foods is absorbed by the body through the small intestine. This absorption is decreased by fibres, calcium, copper, phytate, and phosphate in pulses. In contrast, amino acids and peptides increase zinc absorption. Nearly 99 per cent of the total zinc in the body is stored in cells and the remainder in the plasma and extracellular fluids. Excretion of zinc occurs principally through secretions of the pancreas and intestine.

Functions in the Body

Zinc is needed for a healthy skin and hair, proper healing of wounds, successful pregnancies, and male virility. It plays a vital role in guarding against disease and infection. It is needed to transport vitamin A to the retina. Almost all the enzymes in the body require zinc for their functioning. It has long been known that growth and sexual maturity depend on zinc amongst other things.

Sources

Cereals, nuts and oilseeds are important sources of zinc. Vegetables and fruits contain only a small quantity of zinc.

Rich Sources of Zinc*

Cereals, Pulses & Legumes	mg		mg
		Potatoes	0.5
Bengal gram, whole	6.1	Bitter gourd, white	0.4
Kidney beans	4.5	Cauliflower	0.4
Soya beans, black	4.4	French beans	0.4
Soya beans, white	3.4	Ladies' fingers	0.4
Black gram, whole	3.3	Onions	0.4
Bajra	3.1	Cabbage	0.3
Lentil	3.1	Carrots	0.3
Split black gram	3.0	Cluster beans	0.3
Split green gram	2.8	Colocasia	0.3
Maize, dry	2.8	Spinach	0.3
Wheat, whole	2.7		
Peas	2.3	**Nuts & Oilseeds**	
Jowar	1.6	Cashew nuts	5.9
Barley	1.2	Coconut, dry	5.0
		Mustard seeds	4.8
Vegetables		Groundnuts	3.9
Betel leaves	3.4	Almonds	3.5
Onion stalks	2.2	Walnuts	2.3
Beetroots	0.9		

* Values per 100 g edible portions.

Deficiency Symptoms

Zinc deficiency in the diet has been reported to be the cause of anaemia, retardation in growth, and delayed genital maturation.

Healing and Therapeutic Properties

Oral doses of zinc sulphate may accelerate the healing of chronic skin ulcers and wounds. Patients with these problems have a low content of zinc in the plasma for many weeks despite corticosteroid therapy.

Acne. Zinc seems to offer new promise of help for acne patients. It has shown dramatic results in some cases. Zinc should be taken in therapeutic doses of 50 mg, three times a day. It can be gradually reduced after a noticeable improvement.

Eczema. Zinc has also been found beneficial in the treatment of eczema. Many people with this skin problem have tried and benefitted from zinc supplements. The average dose should be 30 mg a day.

Prostate Disorders. Administration of zinc has been found to be helpful in cases of prostate enlargement. About 30 mg of this mineral should be taken daily in the treatment of these disorders.

Precautions. Excessive intake of zinc can cause loss of iron and copper in the body. Toxicity can result from inhalation of zinc fumes by welders. Inhalation of high concentrations of zinc oxide fumes leads to an acute illness called metal fume fever or brass chills, characterised by fever, chills, excessive salivation, headaches, and a cough.

Airola, Paavo. *How to Get Well*. Arizona: Health Plus Pub., 1974.

Aman. *Medicinal Secrets of Your Food*. Mysore: Indo-American Hospital, N.R. Mohalla, 1985.

Bricklin, Mark. *Natural Home Remedies*. Rodale Press, 1986.

Clark, Linda. *Get Well Naturally*. Reprint. New York: Arco Publishing, 1980.

Clark, Linda. *Stay Young Longer*. Reprint. New York: Jove Publications, 1981.

Davis, Adelle. *Let's Get Well*. U.S.A.: New American Lib., 1972.

Kordel, Lelord. *Health the Easy Way*. Reprint. New York: Award Books, 1976.

Mindell, Earl. *The Vitamin Bible*. Reprint. New Delhi: Allied Publishers, 1983.

Pulunin, Miriam. *Minerals What They are and Why We Need Them*. Wellinborough: Thorsons Publishers Limited, 1979.

Swaminathan, M. *Handbook of Food and Nutrition*. 4th ed. Bangalore: The Bangalore Printing and Publishing Co. Ltd., 1984.

Braunwald, Eugene, Kurt J. Isselbacher, Robert G. Petersdorf, Jean D. Wilson, Joseph B. Martin, and Anthony S. Fauci. *Harrison's Principles of Internal Medicine*. 11th ed. New York: McGraw Hill Book Company, 1988.

Brown, J. A. C., M. B. Bchir. *Pears Medical Encyclopaedia*. Reprint. London: Sphere Books Limited, 1974.

Davidson, Stanley, R. Passmore, J. F. Brock & A. S. Truswell. *Human Nutrition & Dietetics*. 6th ed. Great Britain: The English Language Book Society & Churchill Livingstone, 1975.

Gailaabiz, R. Cheriette, John B. Allreb. *Taking the Fear Out of Eating*. Cambridge University Press, 1992.

Mitchell, Rynbergen, Anderson, and Dibble. *Nutrition in Health and Diseases*. 16th ed. Philadelphia: J. B. Lippincott Co., 1976.

Rao, B.S. Narasinga, Y.G. Deosthale, K.C. Pant. *Nutritive Value of Indian Foods*. Revised reprint. Hyderabad, India: National Institute of Nutrition, ICMR, 1993.

PART III
The Amazing Power of Amino Acid

Rich Sources of Proteins*

Cereals	g
Wheat, germ	29.2
Rice bran	13.5
Panivaragu	12.5
Italian millet	12.3
Wheat flour, whole	12.1
Wheat, whole	11.8
Bajra	11.6
Barley	11.5
Maize, dry	11.1
Jowar	10.4

Pulses & Legumes	g
Soya beans	43.2
Split kesari	28.2
Lentil	25.1
Field beans, dry	24.9
Split green gram	24.5
Cow peas	24.1
Green gram, whole	24.0
Split black gram	24.0
Moth beans	23.6
Kidney beans	22.9

Vegetables	g
Fetid cassia, dried	20.7
Colocasia leaves, dried	13.7
Water chestnut, dry	13.4

Nuts & Oilseeds	g
Groundnut cake	40.9
Water melon seeds	34.1
Groundnuts, roasted	26.2
Garden cress seeds	25.3
Cashewnuts	21.2
Almonds	20.8
Pistachio nuts	19.8
Suflower seeds	19.8
Piyal seeds	19.0
Gingelly seeds	18.3

Fish, Meat & Poultry	g
Beef meal	79.2
Ribbon fish, dried	76.1
Shrimp, small, dried	68.1
Mushi, dried	67.0
Parsey, dried	65.0
Chela, dried	64.8
Chingri, small, dried	62.4
Bombay duck, dried	61.7
Bhagon, dried	61.5
Chingri, goda, dried	60.0
Chicken	25.9
Liver, goat	20.0
Liver, sheep	19.3
Mutton	18.5

Milk & Milk Products	g
Skimmed milk powder, cow's milk	38.0
Wholemilk powder, cow's milk	25.8
Cheese	24.1
Khoa, skimmed milk, buffalo's	22.3
Khoa, wholemilk, cow's	20.0
Cottage cheese, cow's milk	18.3

* Values in g per 100 g edible portions.

An amino acid can be defined as any of a large group of organic compounds which represent the end products of protein breakdown. All proteins are made up of amino acids. Life without protein is not possible. Growth, development, and function depend upon protein, which, in turn, depends upon the correct availability of amino acids. When we take protein it must first be broken down into amino acids before it can be absorbed by the body. This takes place in the small bowel. From there, the fragments of protein are carried to the liver by the bloodstream, where they are stored for future use. When needed by the body, these fragments are finally recombined into the type of protein needed by each particular kind of cell.

All amino acids comprise a carbon atom, an amino group(containing nitrogen), and a carboxyl group. Plants synthesise amino acids from three sources: the soil which supplies the necessary nitrogen and sulphur, water which provides oxygen and hydrogen, and atmospheric carbon dioxide which supplies carbon and oxygen. With the help of synthesising bacteria and fungi, plants unite these elements into amino acids. Animals cannot synthesise amino acids from these basic elements but derive them from the ingestion of plants. Thus the primary source of all proteins, including meat and fish, is the vegetable kingdom.

The mere division of nutrients into groups such as vitamins, minerals, and amino acids does not mean that they are effective individually. An interrelationship exists among the three nutrients, and they may lose their efficiency if any one of the nutrients is not present in its optimum quantity. All proteins are not nutritionally equivalent. This difference in nutritional value is based on the amino acid composition of different proteins. This has led to the concept of Essential Amino Acids (EAA) and Non-Essential Amino Acids(NEAA). An essential amino acid is indispensable: it cannot be sythesised in the body in adequate amounts to meet the requirements for protein synthesis. Taking a diet which does not contain adequate amounts of any of the essential amino acids, leads to negative nitrogen balance. This can occur even when the total dietary intake of protein is apparently adequate.

By contrast, non-essential amino acids can be omitted from the diet, so long as it contains adequate amounts of total protein. This is so because the body can manufacture them in adequate amounts to meet the needs for protein synthesis. Non-essential amino acids are, therefore, dispensable.

There are 23 amino acids. Eight of them are strictly dietary essentials and cannot be synthesised at all by the body. These are isoleucine, leucine, lysine, methionine, phenylalanine, threonine, tryptophan, and valine. In addition to these strictly essential amino acids, two other amino acids, namely, arginine and histidine, are essential for infants and young persons, as the capacity for their synthesis in the body is not adequate to meet the needs for growth.

In addition to the ten essential amino acids mentioned above, there are 13 non-essential amino acids. They are proline, carnitine, tyrosine, glutamic acid and glutamine, cysteine and cystine, glycine, alanine, b-alanine, aspartic acid, taurine, ornithine, citrulline, and gama-aminobutyric acid(GABA). Under special conditions, the demand for some of the non-essential amino acids may be greater than the synthetic capacity, and therefore, they too can become dietary essentials.

About 75 per cent of the amino acids entering the bloodstream through the liver from the gastro-intestinal tract after a meal, are metabolised in the liver, and only about 25 per cent enter the general circulation. Out of the intake of amino acids in excess of immediate requirements, upto 50 per cent are catabolised for energy-yielding metabolism, and non-essential amino acids that have not been ingested in adequate amounts are synthesised for transport to other tissues. The nitrogen from this amino acid catabolism is not excreted immediately, but a considerable amount of urea is recirculated through the gastro-intestinal tract and reabsorbed as ammonia. This enables the synthesis of non-essential amino acids from suitable metabolic intermediates to continue when there is no dietary intake. Under normal conditions human beings excrete about 3 g of amino acids in the urine every day.

Amino acid deficiency may be the result of protein malnutrition. Such deficiency is generally associated with a faulty diet, failure to digest or absorb adequately, stress conditions, infection, trauma, use of drugs, deficiency of other nutrients such as vitamins and minerals, and dysfunctions connected with the ageing process. Since amino acids perform such a major role in the structure and function of the body, in both health maintenance and disease, the importance of available tests to assess their relative presence cannot be underestimated. Much research has been done in recent years. Tests not only disclose the nutritional and metabolic status of the patient, they also discover the effects of factors such as stress, trauma, and drugs.

The deficiency conditions resulting from any of these causes can be corrected by supplementation of appropriate amino acids.

The various functions of the essential and frequently investigated non-essential amino acids, their deficiency symptoms, and their therapeutic uses are discussed in subsequent chapters.

Increases Male Sexual Vitality

Arginine is an essential amino acid. It is obtained from food during the growth period, but can subsequently be manufactured by the body. Eighty per cent of the male seminal fluid is made of arginine, hence, it is known as the 'fatherhood' amino acid. At present there is no accurate scientific evidence about the recommended daily allowance of Arginine.

Arginine is needed for the formation of proteins such as collagen and elastin, and vital substances such as haemoglobin, insulin, and glucagon.

Functions in the Body

Arginine is essential for normal growth and proper functioning of the immune system in the body. It is broken down into ornithine and urea and is, therefore, a vital part of the urea cycle in the liver, which is the main route of detoxification and elimination of urea.

Sources

Major food sources of arginine are peanuts, cashew nuts, piyal seeds, water melon seeds, and walnuts. This amino acid is found in most vegetables, especially green and root vegetables. Arginine exists in a free state in such plants as garlic and ginseng.

Deficiency Symptoms

Lack of arginine reduces the sex impulse and can cause impotence. A prolonged deficiency is not only harmful to the immunological system but can also result in disordered carbohydrate metabolism.

Healing and Therapeutic Properties

Arginine is useful in some cases of male sterility. A supplementary use of arginine minimises post-wound weight loss and accelerates wound healing. Animal experiments have indicated that an extra intake of dietary arginine brings down cholesterol levels in the blood, atherosclerosis, and narrowing of the blood vessels. An increased intake in the diet can also lead to an increase in weight and muscle mass. The dosages suggested in this particular programme are 2 g on an empty stomach before retiring, and 2 g on an empty stomach one hour prior to vigorous exercise.

Precautions. Several weeks of supplementation in mature adults may cause reversible thickening and coarsening of the skin. Arginine is contraindicated in cases of herpes simplex infections according to a number of authorities. Foods rich in arginine should therefore be avoided by patients with such viral infections.

For Tissue Growth and Repair

Histidine is regarded as an essential amino acid during the period of growth. However as healthy adults are capable of synthesising it according to their requirements, it is termed a non-essential amino acid in adult life. This amino acid may also be required in the diet during old age and in those suffering from degenerative diseases. Histidine is metabolised into histamine, an important physiological substance which is normally freely present in the intestine.

Recommended
Daily Allowance*
Infants   33 mg

Functions in the Body

Histidine is essential for growth and the repair of human tissues. It is necessary for the conversion of glucose into glycogen in the liver. Histidine converted into histamine stimulates the secretion of hydrochloric acid in the stomach.

Sources

Histidine is found in fruits such as bananas and grapes, meat and poultry, and milk and milk products. It is also found in root vegetables and all green vegetables, though in lesser quantities.

Deficiency Symptoms

A deficiency of histidine can cause pain in the bony joints. A low urine concentration of histidine has been reported to accompany rheumatoid arthritis.

* Value per kg of body weight.

Healing and Therapeutic Properties

Taken orally, histidine is likely to depress the pain of rheumatoid arthritis. Professor Gerber of Downstate Medical Center, New York, utilises between 1 g and 6 g daily in arthritic patients.

Histidine helps to dilate the blood vessels and has, therefore, been found beneficial in the treatment of cardio-circulatory disorders.

The release of histamine from body stores is considered a prerequisite for sexual arousal. Hence histidine supplementation may prove helpful in this regard.

Histidine has also been found to be beneficial in allergic conditions, in the treatment of anaemia, and disorders of the auditory nerve.

Precautions. Taken orally, histidine has a tendency to stimulate hydrochloric acid secretion in the stomach. Thus persons who already suffer from overabundance of acid in the stomach and those who have ulcers should avoid taking pure histidine.

Stimulates Essential Hormones

Isoleucine is an essential amino acid: that is, it is not formed in the body and hence, must be present in the diet. Along with leucine and valine, it is important in human metabolism as an energy-yielding source.

Recommended Daily Allowance*	
Men	12 mg
Women	12 mg
Children	28 mg
Infants	80 mg

Functions in the Body

Isoleucine is essential for the production and maintenance of body proteins. It also regulates metabolism and the functioning of the thymus gland in the neck, spleen, and pituitary glands. It is useful in the formation of haemoglobin.

Sources

Rich sources of isoleucine are eggs, chicken, pork, mutton, pulses, soya beans, cottage cheese, milk, piyal seeds, cashew nuts, and cereal grains.

Healing and Therapeutic Properties

Isoleucine is one of a group of amino acids found deficient in persons who are ill. The recommended therapeutic dose of this amino acid is between 240 mg and 360 mg daily. Hence this must be given in combination with the other amino acids that are found lacking.

---

* Values per kg of body weight.

Boosts Energy Levels

Leucine is an essential amino acid, and along with isoleucine and valine, plays an important role in energy production in the body.

Recommended Daily Allowance*	
Men	16 mg
Women	16 mg
Children	42 mg
Infants	128 mg

Functions in the Body

Leucine regulates protein metabolism in the body. The availability of leucine is especially important in controlling the net synthesis of protein.

Sources

The major sources of leucine are whole grains and milk and milk products. Eggs, pork, beef, chicken, pulses, soya beans, and leafy vegetables are good sources of leucine.

Healing and Therapeutic Properties

Therapeutically, leucine as well as isoleucine and valine can be used as a means of minimising protein loss in patients undergoing surgery.

Precautions. In some studies, it has been found that dietary excess of leucine may be a precipitating factor in developing pellagra.

---

* Values per kg of body weight.

The Anti-Virus Factor

Lysine is an essential amino acid which cannot be synthesised in the body. It is therefore essential that the diet should contain adequate quantities of it. Cereal proteins such as rice, wheat, oats, millet, and sesame seeds are deficient in lysine. Vitamin C has a protective effect on the body levels of lysine.

Recommended Daily Allowance*	
Men	12 mg
Women	12 mg
Child en	44 mg
Infants	97 mg

Functions in the Body

Lysine inhibits the proliferation of viruses. Along with vitamin C, zinc, and vitamin A, it helps in eliminating virus infections. Since vitamin C protects this amino acid in the body, lysine with vitamin C has a much stronger anti-virus effect than if either is used separately.

Sources

The main sources of lysine are leafy vegetables, pulses and legumes, meat, poultry, milk and milk products, and ripe fruits.

Deficiency Symptoms

The insufficient intake of lysine in the diet can lead to a poor appetite, reduction in body weight, anaemia, and a reduced ability to concentrate. It may also cause headaches, dizziness, and nausea. Lysine deficiency in the body has also been associated with pneumonia,

---

* Values per kg of body weight.

nephrosis, and acidosis, as well as with malnutrition and rickets in children.

Healing and Therapeutic Properties

Lysine is considered to be a natural remedy for cold sores, shingles, and genital herpes. It exercises beneficial effects in viral-related diseases, particularly herpes simplex. During episodes of acute herpes, a minimum of 1,500 mg of lysine and at least one gram of vitamin C should be taken daily.

Lysine is used therapeutically to assist gastric function and appetite. It thus helps to enhance the growth of children. The therapeutic dosage recommended for this purpose is 500 mg-1,500 mg daily.

Protects the Liver

Methionine is an essential amino acid. A sulphur-containing amino acid, it is required in the body for making nucleic acid and collagen, and protein synthesis. The body can make cysteine, another amino

Recommended Daily Allowance*	
Men	10 mg
Women	10 mg
Children	22 mg
Infants	45 mg

acid, from methionine but not vice versa. It can also make choline, a vitamin of the B complex group, in the body with the aid of vitamin B_{12} and folacin, provided the diet is high in protein. It acts as an antioxidant, and as such, removes harmful free radicals from the body.

Functions in the Body

Of all the amino acids, methionine is of key importance for the health of the liver. It protects the liver from fatty degeneration. The cysteine that it forms prevents the destruction of the liver cells. This amino acid helps dissolve cholesterol and assimilates fat. It is required by the pancreas, lymph nodes, and the spleen, and is essential for the synthesis of haemoglobin. It is necessary for the maintenance of normal body weight and also helps to maintain the proper nitrogen balance in the body. Studies show that methionine and choline prevent tumour formation.

---

* Values per kg of body weight.

Sources

Rich sources of methionine are whole grains. It is also found in meat and poultry, and milk and milk products. Leafy vegetables, peaches and grapes also contain methionine.

Deficiency Symptoms

The deficiency of methionine can ultimately lead to chronic rheumatic fever in children, hardening of the liver(cirrhosis), and nephritis of the kidneys. According to the nutritional expert, Adelle Davis, deficiency of methionine can be the cause of choline deficiency, as it can lead to retention of fat in the liver.

Healing and Therapeutic Properties

Methionine is considered to be one of the body's most powerful detoxifying agents. It detoxifies histamine when levels of the latter are high in schizophrenic patients.

The therapeutic dosage of methionine varies from 200 mg-1,000 mg daily. This amino acid has also been found valuable in cases of high blood cholesterol, as it brings down the blood cholesterol levels.

For Weight Control

Phenylalanine is an essential amino acid since other amino acids are formed from it in the body. Along with tyrosine, it provides raw material from which the body makes the hormones adrenaline and thyroxine. The body can also convert phenylalanine to tyrosine but not vice versa.

Recommended Daily Allowance*	
Men	16 mg
Women	16 mg
Children	22 mg
Infants	132 mg

Functions in the Body

Phenylalanine is effective for weight control because of its effect on thyroid secretion. It also plays an important role in the control of appetite. If taken before meals, it suppresses the appetite substantially. This amino acid is also essential for the efficient functioning of the kidneys and the bladder.

Sources

Phenylalanine is found in abundance in curd, milk, cottage cheese, pulses and legumes, poultry, piyal seeds, groundnuts, pistachio nuts, almonds, leafy vegetables, and whole grains.

Deficiency Symptoms

Deficiency of phenylalanine can lead to a variety of symptoms including bloodshot eyes, cataract, and several behavioural changes, such as psychotic and schizophrenic behaviour.

---

* Values per kg of body weight.

Healing and Therapeutic Properties

Phenylalanine has many therapeutic uses. It is considered beneficial in the treatment of obesity and is being successfully employed as an appetite suppressant for this condition. It has been demonstrated that in the intestinal tract, the amino acids tryptophan and phenylalanine trigger the release of cholycystokinin (CCK) which induces satiety, and a termination of eating.

An intake of half a teaspoon of phenylalanine powder 30 minutes before each meal, can lead to a loss of as much as 100 to 200 g of weight a day.

The other positive effects noticed after 24–48 hours of taking phenylalanine are a feeling of greater alertness, an increase in sexual interest, and memory enhancement. It diminishes depressant feelings, if any. The depressant states are generally relieved within a few days by taking 100 mg-500 mg of 1-phenylalanine per day.

Precautions. Caution should be observed in the use of phenylalanine in hypertensive individuals. Low doses of around 100 mg daily should be taken by anyone with suspected high blood pressure, and a check should be kept on pressure levels. Phenylalanine should not be taken by those who are taking drugs such as Aldomet for high blood pressure.

Therapy for Mental Illness

Threonine is an essential amino acid. Along with lysine, it is deficient in most foodgrains, but present in most pulses. A combination of foodgrains and pulses provides an adequate supply of these amino acids in a vegetarian diet.

Recommended Daily Allowance*	
Men	8 mg
Women	8 mg
Children	28 mg
Infants	63 mg

Threonine is necessary for the development and proper functioning of the brain, particularly in children. It also has a powerful anti-convulsive effect.

Sources

Threonine is found in poultry, pork, and leafy vegetables. Whole grains, pulses, nuts, apples, peaches, and figs also contain threonine.

Deficiency Symptoms

Deficiency of threonine can result in irritability in children.

Healing and Therapeutic Properties

Cheraksin Williams lists threonine, along with most of the B vitamins, magnesium, ascorbic acid, iodine, potassium, tryptophan, lysine, inositol, and glutamic acid as being essential in the prevention and treatment of mental illness.

Threonine is said to be very useful in indigestion and intestinal malfunctions, as well as prevention of excessive fat in the liver. A fatty liver, resulting from a low-protein diet, can be corrected by threonine.

* Values per kg of body weight.

Sleep-Inducing

Out of all essential amino acids, the most research has been carried out by nutritional researchers on tryptophan. It is also known as a sleep-inducing amino acid.

Recommended Daily Allowance*		
Men	3	mg
Women	3	mg
Children	4	mg
Infants	19	mg

Functions in the Body

Tryptophan plays a significant role in the synthesis of one of the B complex group of vitamins called niacin or nicotinic acid. In the human system, an average of about 1 mg of niacin is formed from 60 mg of dietary tryptophan.

This amino acid is also essential for blood clotting and formation of digestive juices. It induces sleep and relaxes the nervous system. It wards off signs of premature ageing, such as cataract of the eyes, baldness, deterioration of sex gland functioning, and malformation of tooth enamel.

Tryptophan is also important as a major precursor of the transmitter amine, serotinin, in the central nervous system.

Sources

Generally all seeds, nuts, and most vegetables contain tryptophan. The best sources of this amino acid, however, are bajra, barley, finger millet, colocasia, sweet potatoes, cashew nuts, mangoes, papayas, and milk.

---

* Values per kg of body weight.

Deficiency Symptoms

The failure of absorption of tryptophan in cases of intestinal disorders can cause increased sensitivity to light, leading to excessive scaling of the skin on exposure to the sun. A deficiency of tryptophan and niacin causes pellagra, a deficiency disease characterised by three Ds: dermatitis, diarrhoea, dementia.

Healing and Therapeutic Properties

Tryptophan can be used as a safe and effective food remedy for certain ailments, especially insomnia and emotional complaints.

Insomnia. Tryptophan is a precursor of serotinin which is regarded as an effective sleep-inducing agent. Researches have been carried out by Dr. E. Hartmann of Boston State Hospital on the therapeutic effectiveness of tryptophan in insomnia. He has reported: 'In our studies we found that a dose of one gram of tryptophan would cut down the time it takes to fall asleep from twenty to ten minutes. Its great advantage is that not only do you get to sleep sooner, but you do so without distortions in sleep patterns that are produced by most sleeping pills.' It has been found that tryptophan is an effective hypnotic when administered at any time of the day, and that it significantly reduces the time of onset of sleep without affecting the various stages of sleep.

Aches and Pains. Tryptophan is regarded as a natural painkiller. A study at the Department of Neurology at the University of Tampere in Finland, indicates that this amino acid has potential as a pain-reducing agent.

Emotional Complaints. Research has shown that there is an inverse relationship between tryptophan consumption and emotional complaints. Increasing the tryptophan intake decreases the number and severity of such complaints. Studies carried out on a group of 66 individuals who were given tryptophan supplementation for several months indicated that those who had increased their intake from 1,001 mg per day to an average of 1,331 mg per day, showed a remarkable decrease in the number of psychological complaints, whereas those who had not altered their tryptophan intake showed no change.

Tryptophan is best taken between meals with a low-protein food such as fruit juice or bread. One to three grams a day seems to be the range favoured by most researchers.

Tooth Decay. A recent experiment has shown that tryptophan can prevent tooth decay. According to a report by Naomi C. Turner of Radcliffe College, this amino acid offers distinct promise as a preventive for dental decay. This is based on the finding that it slows down the rate of starch decomposition. It was previously noted that there was a definite relationship between tooth decay and the rate of starch decomposition. Persons with twenty or more cavities were found to produce saliva which decomposed starchy food very rapidly. Persons with little or no tooth decay produced saliva which decomposed starch very slowly. Thus, if tryptophan in some form(in a toothpaste, as a chewing gum, even mixed with starchy food) could slow down the rate of carbohydrate decomposition, then in all likelihood, the rate of tooth decay could also be greatly lessened.

Recent research by Dr G. Chowinard of Mc Gill University, Montreal, indicates that the functional usefulness of tryptophan is enhanced by the concurrent supplementation of nicotinic acid. The ratio suggested is two parts of tryptophan to one part of nicotinic acid.

Precautions. The use of supplementary tryptophan should be avoided during pregnancy.

Prevents Nervous Disorders

Valine is an essential amino acid which is considered important for body growth. It is needed for the proper performance of the nervous system; an adequate intake prevents nervous and digestive disorders.

Recommended Daily Allowance*	
Men	14 mg
Women	14 mg
Children	25 mg
Infants	89 mg

Sources

The main food sources of valine are leafy vegetables, finger millet, rice and other cereals, kidney beans and other legumes and pulses, piyal seeds, pistachio and cashew nuts, and peaches. Poultry and milk contain a large amount of valine.

Deficiency Symptoms

The lack of valine makes a person sensitive to touch and sound.

Healing and Therapeutic Properties

W. Borrman, a nutrition researcher, describes valine as helpful in disorders of the muscles, mental and emotional upsets, insomnia, and nervousness. Valine intake as a part of the amino-acid combination of phenylalanine-valine-methionine-tryptophan in the ratio of 3:2:2:1, taken in 4 g doses prior to meals, results in decreased food intake in 50 per cent of obese women.

Precautions. Excess of valine leads to symptoms such as hallucinations and a sensation of insects crawling over the skin.

---

* Values per kg of body weight.

Alanine

Alanine is a non-essential amino acid. It plays an important function in the metabolism of the essential amino acid tryptophan and the vitamin pyridoxine.

In cases of hypoglycaemia, alanine may be used for the production of glucose so that the blood glucose levels stabilise in the long term.

B-Alanine

B-Alanine is a non-essential amino acid. It is the only naturally occurring b-amino acid. It is found in the brain, and is useful in the synthesis of pantothenic acid(vitamin B_5).

Asparagine and Aspartic Acid

Aspartic acid is a non-essential amino acid which is crucial for general body metabolism. It is found in plants, especially in sprouting seeds. In protein it exists mainly as asparagine.

Asparagine is of therapeutic use in brain and neurological imbalances. This amino acid increases the resistance to fatigue, thereby stepping up the stamina of athletes. It enhances the smooth functioning of the liver.

Carnitine

Like Taurine, carnitine is a non-essential amino acid which is present in muscle and organ meats, and synthesised in the liver. The supply of carnitine depends upon the ingestion of some essential amino acids, particularly, lysine and methionine. An adequate amount of vitamin C is also necessary. Men seem to have a greater need for carnitine than women.

Healing and Therapeutic Properties. Carnitine plays an important function in the metabolism of fat and the reduction of triglycerides in the body. One to three grams of carnitine should be administered daily for the required oxidation of triglycerides, especially when there is poor hand and foot co-ordination, myocardial infarction, and kidney disease.

Carnitine is also a useful supplement in cases of muscular dystrophy and cardiac ischemia.

Citrulline

Citrulline is found mainly in the liver and is a major component of the urea cycle. It is found in abundance in plant foods such as onion and garlic.

This non-essential amino acid is useful for detoxification of ammonia and in the treatment of fatigue. A precursor to the essential amino acids arginine and ornithine, citrulline can influence the production of the growth hormone.

Cysteine and Cystine

Cystine is a sulphur-containing, non-essential amino acid. It is a stable form of the sulphur-rich amino acid cysteine. The body is capable of converting one to the other as required. They can be thought of as the same in metabolic terms.

The metabolic steps of the formation of these two amino acids are from methionine→ cystathionine→ cysteine→ cystine. In chronic diseases, it appears that the formation of cysteine from methionine is prevented. It is therefore essential to restore adequate levels of cysteine or cystine in such cases.

Functions in the Body. Cystine provides resistance to the body against harmful effects by building up white blood-cell activity. It is essential for the proper functioning of the skin and helps in recovery from surgery. It promotes the formation of carotene which helps hair growth. The flexibility of the skin, as well as the texture, is influenced by cysteine as it has the ability to protect collagen, the connective tissue protein.

Cystine has been shown to protect the body against damage caused by alcohol and cigarette smoking. One report states that not only is it effective in preventing the side-effects of drinking, such as a hangover, but it prevents liver and brain damage as well. It also reduces lung damage such as emphysema, resulting from smoking.

Sources. Cystine ia available in whole grains, soya beans, and leafy vegetables. Pistachio nuts, bananas, dates, meat, eggs, and milk all contain cystine.

Healing and Therapeutic Properties. Cystine is used in the treatment of skin diseases, for low count of white blood cells, and in some cases, for anaemia.

Kidney Stones. Some stones in the kidney are made up of uric acid or the amino acid cystine. To prevent the formation of such stones, large amounts of fruits and vegetables, especially citrus fruits, are recommended. They help to produce an alkaline urine which prevents crystal formation in these amino acids.

Excessive loss of cystine in the urine is said to be a hereditary disorder. A few cases have been helped by being given large amounts of choline.

Obesity. Dr H. Ghadimi, Chairman of the Nutrition Committee at Nassau Country Medical Centre in New York, uses cysteine supplements to treat his patients suffering from obesity. He considers that there is a link between obesity and overproduction of insulin, and that cysteine supplements taken along with vitamin C at the end of a meal, somehow neutralise some of the excess insulin which is responsible for fat production. He regards this amino acid as anti-cancer and anti-ageing, and claims that like vitamin C, cysteine protects the body from damage by oxidants.

Precautions. Accumulation of free cystine in the body tissues can lead to a rare disease known as cystinosis. This results in the appearance of cystine crystals in the cornea, conjuctiva; bone marrow, lymph nodes, leukocytes, and internal organs.

Persons with diabetic tendencies should not use large supplemental doses of cysteine except under medical supervision, as it is capable of inactivating insulin by reducing certain disulphide bonds which determine its structure.

In order to avoid the conversion of cysteine to cystine, with possible consequences of the formation of kidney or bladder stones, an intake of three times the dose of vitamin C has been suggested to accompany the taking of cysteine supplementally.

Gama-Aminobutyric acid(GABA)

Gama-aminobutyric acid(GABA) is a non-essential amino acid derived from glutamic acid. It regulates the transmission of chemical impulses in the central nervous system and is, therefore, essential for brain metabolism.

Used in the treatment of epilepsy and hypertension, it induces calmness and tranquility. It is also useful in reducing problems related to an enlarged prostrate, by stimulating the release of the hormone prolactin from the pituitary gland. The doses recommended are 20 to 40 mg daily, dissolved under the tongue. This, however, should only be taken under medical guidance.

Glutamine and Glutamic Acid

Glutamine is a non-essential amino acid. J. Bland, a nutrition researcher, however, suggests that under certain conditions it may become a 'contingency nutrient', and, therefore, be considered essential. He points out that glutamine is synthesised in certain tissues for use in others. Glutamic acid can be synthesised from a number of amino acids.

Functions in the Body. Known as the 'sobriety amino acid', glutamine is involved in two important roles. Along with glucose, it is fuel for the brain cells. The second function of glutamine is to act as a detoxifier of ammonia from the brain. As it picks up ammonia, glutamic acid is reconverted to its original form of glutamine. Glutamic acid also plays an important role in the metabolism of ammonia.

Deficiency Symptoms. Glutamine deficiencies are seldom seen. However, a contingency status may be reached through extensive demand in relation to genetic factors which lead to an inadequate synthesis in the body.

As the brain is able to store relatively small quantities of glucose, it is dependent upon glutamic acid. The shortage of glutamine or glutamic acid in the brain results in brain damage or dullness of brain due to excess ammonia.

Healing and Therapeutic Properties. Glutamine is considered beneficial in the treatment of alcoholism. It plays a protective role in the body's relationship with alcohol. An amount of two to four grams glutamine taken daily, is the suggested treatment for alcohol problems.

Dr Bernard Rimland of the Institute for Child Behaviour has successfully improved behavioural problems in children by nutritional means, which include glutamic acid as a major component.

Other noted areas in which glutamine can be used beneficially are depression, IQ improvement in mentally deficient children, healing of peptic ulcers, epilepsy in children, and schizophrenia.

Glutathione

Glutathione is a naturally occurring tripeptide consisting of three amino acids — cysteine, glutamic acid, and glycine. It is of great use in the prevention and treatment of many degenerative diseases. It accomplishes this by preventing and slowing down the activity of free radicals which suppress the body's natural immunity and hasten the ageing process.

Liver damage caused by excessive intake of alcohol is also prevented by glutathione.

Glycine

Another non-essential amino acid, glycine, is a major constituent of the liver-detoxifying compound glutathione, along with cysteine and glutamic acid.

Research on human beings indicates that glycine enhances the secretion of acid in the stomach.

Ornithine

Ornithine is a non-essential amino acid. It is an important constituent of the urea cycle. It is also the precursor of other amino acids such as citrulline, glutamic acid, and proline. It enhances the functioning of the liver and is used to treat hepatic coma.

Some researchers maintain that the growth hormone is released when a supplement of 1-2 g of ornithine is taken on a relatively empty stomach at bedtime. They also claim that the immune system is thus stimulated, improving the immunity to bacteria, viruses, and tumours. However, there is still no proven validity of a long-term impact of this claim. Also, schizophrenics are strongly advised against the use of ornithine.

Proline

Proline is a non-essential amino acid. It is one of the main components of collagen, the cementing substance that binds and supports the cells.

Research seems to indicate the usefulness of proline in the healing of wounds. Its effectiveness is enhanced when combined with vitamin C. Supplementation is advised in cases of persistent soft tissue strains, hypermobile joints, and in lax tissues associated with ageing. The therapeutic dose advised is 500 mg to 1,000 mg daily, in combination with vitamin C.

Taurine

Taurine is a non-essential amino acid. It is manufactured in the body and is present in animal protein. Its synthesis occurs in the human body with the help of the amino acids methionine, cysteine, and vitamin B_6. Women seem to require a higher dietary intake of taurine, since the female hormone estradiol supresses the formation of taurine in the liver.

An important function of taurine is its role as a neurotransmitter. It also maintains the correct composition of bile and the solubility of cholesterol.

Healing and Therapeutic Properties. Studies have shown that taurine concentrations in the brain are four times more in developing brains than in adult ones. Trials on human beings have proved that taurine has an anticonvulsive effect. During epileptic attacks, the serum levels of over half the amino acids are lowered. One gram of taurine, taken daily, followed by daily doses of not more than 500 mg, further reduced to 50-100 mg a day, is more effective than taking higher doses.

Taurine also protects the heart muscle when there is calcium and potassium loss from the body. Supplementation of taurine is said to improve IQ levels in children suffering from Down's syndrome.

Heart disorders, physical or emotional stress, metabolic disorders, high alcohol consumption, and zinc deficiency are factors that can result in high levels of taurine being excreted in the urine.

Tyrosine

Tyrosine is a non-essential amino acid and is popularly called the anti-stress amino acid. It is derived from phenylalanine, an essential amino acid. It is an essential component of the thyroid hormone.

Functions in the Body. Along with phenylalanine, tyrosine provides raw material from which the body makes the hormones thyroxine and adrenaline. The pigment of the skin and hair, melanin, is also derived from tyrosine.

The supplement may be divided into three separate doses per day. When tyrosine is taken, a supplement of valine(an essential amino acid) should not be taken, as valine may block the entry of tyrosine to the brain.

Sources. Rice, leafy vegetables, curd, cheese, and milk contain generous amounts of tyrosine.

Deficiency Symptoms. Deficiency of tyrosine can lead to low body temperature, low blood pressure, and a restless feeling in the legs.

Healing and Therapeutic Properties. Brain tyrosine levels are most conveniently raised by ingestion of pure tyrosine, with a high carbohydrate meal. There is evidence that small doses of tyrosine hasten the transmission of impulses in the brain.

Dr Richard Wurtman who conducted experiments on the use of tyrosine says, 'Supplemented tyrosine may be useful therapeutically in persons exposed chronically to stress.'

Tyrosine is also beneficial in the treatment of depression. Research has established this amino acid to be effective in the management and control of depression in conjunction with glutamine, tryptophan, niacin, and vitamin B_6.

Bender, David A. *Amino Acid Metabolism.* 2nd ed. Great Britain: John Willey and Sons, 1985.

Chaitow, Leon. *Amino Acids in Therapy.* New York: Thomsons Publishers Ltd., 1985.

Dairs, Adelle. *Let's Get Well.* USA: New American Library, 1972.

Kordel, Lelord. *Health the Easy Way.* New York: Award Books, 1976.

Braunwald, Eugene, Kurt J. Isselbacher, Robert G. Petersdorf, Jean D. Wilson, Joseph B. Martin, and Anthony S. Fauci. *Harrison's Principles of Internal Medicine.* 11th ed. New York: McGraw Hill Book Company, 1988.

Mitchell, Rynbergen, Anderson, and Dibble. *Nutrition in Health and Diseases.* 16th ed. Philadelphia: J.B. Lippincott Company, 1976.

Rao, B.S. Narasingha, Y.G. Deosthale, K.C. Pant. *Nutritive Value of Indian Foods.* Revised and updated reprint. Hyderabad, India: National Institute of Nutrition, ICMR, 1993.

Acidosis. Excessive acid in the blood.

Alopecia. Baldness.

Amine. A molecule having a nitrogen element.

Aneurysm. A swelling produced in a blood vessel due to weakness in its wall.

Anorexia. Loss of appetite.

Arteriosclerosis. Narrowing of the blood vessels.

Autointoxication. Toxins being produced in the body.

Beriberi. Inflammation of the nerves due to vitamin B_1 shortage.

Cadmium. A soft, bluish-white metallic element.

Carcinogens. Any substance producing cancer.

Catabolised. Used up for the production of energy.

Cation. A negatively charged particle.

Cerebral thrombosis. Blockage of the brain blood vessels.

Chylomicrons. Spherules of fat.

Collagen. A cementing substance in-between the cells of the body; its derangement causes many bodily diseases.

Emphysenia. Enlargement of air spaces in the lungs.

Epithelial. Cells lining inner walls of body's hollow organs.

Glucagon. A hormone produced in the pancreas which aids the breakdown of glycogen.

Haemosiderosis. Impregnation of a tissue with the iron-containing portion of haemoglobin.

Herpes simplex. A sexually transmitted viral infection, usually involving the genital organs.

Hydrolysed. The breaking down of fats into fatty acids.

Hypercalcaemia. An excess of calcium in the blood.

Hypertrophy. Enlargement of a tissue or an organ.

Jejenium. The first part of the small intestine.

Keratinise. Hardening of the skin.

Lecithin. A complex fat found in various body tissues, more particularly in the brain and nerves.

Leum. The second part of the small intestine.

Metabolism. A chemical process in a living organism, resulting in energy production.

Mitochondria. The energy-supplying part of a cell.

Myocardial infarction. Destruction of a part of the heart muscle for lack of blood supply.

Myoglobin. An oxygen-carrying protein containing iron present in the muscles.

Myxoedema. A diminished functioning of the thyroid, causing a slowing down in all functions of the body.

Necrosis. Destruction of a tissue.

Nephritis. Inflammation of the kidneys.

Nephrosis. A pathological condition of the kidney which leads to loss of albumin in the urine.

Neurasthenia. Weakness of the nerves.

Neuritis. Inflammation of the nerves.

Oedema. Swelling with fluid.

Osmotic. Tendency of a fluid to pass through a membrane.

Osteomalacia. A disorder in which bones become soft.

Oxalic acid. A kind of acid leading to production of stones.

Parathyroid glands. Hormonal glands in the neck which regulate calcium metabolism in the body.

Phytic acid. A kind of acid produced in the intestines after incomplete absorption of lentils.

Polyneuritis. Inflammation of several nerves at a time.

Porphyria. The presence of excessive porphyrins in the blood which cause skin rashes and mental symptoms.

Seborrhoea. A condition which arises due to over-production of sebum(a kind of fat) in the skin.

Sprue. An intestinal disorder due to malabsorption of food.

Thymus. A hormone-producing gland present in front of the thyroid; very active in the foetus or during infancy.

Vasodilator. A substance causing dilation of blood vessels.

Xeropthalmia. Dryness of eyes, due to lack of tear production.

VITAMIN, MINERAL & AMINO ACID SUPPLEMENTS

The following is the list of brand names of vitamins, minerals and amino acids supplements available in India. The names of the manufacturers are given in the brackets. These supplements are available at most chemist shops. In some cases a doctor's prescription may be required.

Trade Names	Composition	Form
Vitamin A		
AQUASOL A (USV)	Vit. A	Cap.
ADEXOLIN (Glaxo)	Vit. A, D	Cap.
AROVIT (Piramal HC)	Vit. A	Tab./Drp./Inj.
ROVIGON (Piramal HC)	Vit. A, E	Tab.
Vitamin B$_1$		
BENALGIS (Franco Indian)	Vit. B$_1$	Tab.
BENEURON (Franco Indian)	Vit. B$_1$	Cap..
BERIN (Glaxo)	Vit. B$_1$	Tab./Inj.
Vitamin B$_2$		
LIPABOL (Cadila)	Vit. B$_2$	Tab.
Vitamin B$_6$		
B-LONG (Elder)	Vit. B$_6$	Tab.
PYRICONTIN (Modi Mundi Pharma)	Vit. B$_6$	Tab.
Vitamin B$_9$		
FOLIK (Synokem)	Vit. B$_9$	Tab.
FOLVITE (Cyanamid)	Vit. B$_9$	Tab.
Vitamin B$_{12}$		
MACRABIN (Glaxo)	Vit. B$_{12}$	Inj.

1. The abbreviations used in the table are as follows: Cap.: Capsule, Drp.: Drops, Inj.: Injection, Liq.: Liquid, Pdr.: Powder, Prls.: Pearls, Sac.: Sachet, Sol.: Solution, Susp.: Suspension, Syr.: Syrup, Tab.: Tablet

Vitamin C

CEBION (Merck)	Vit. C	Tab.
CECON (Abbott)	Vit. C	Drp.
CELIN (Glaxo)	Vit. C	Tab.
CITRAVITE (Pharmed)	Vit. C	Tab.
LIMCEE (Sarabhai)	Vit. C	Tab.
REDOXON (Roche)	Vit. C	Tab./Inj.
SORVICIN (East India)	Vit. C	Tab./Drp.
SUKCEE (IDPL)	Vit. C	Tab./Drp.
TILDOXON (Tablets India)	Vit. C	Inj.

Vitamin D

ALPHA D3 (Biddle Sawyer)	Vit. D	Cap.
ARACHITOL (Duphar)	Vit. D	Inj.
CALCIROL (Cadila)	Vit. D	Sac.
ONE ALPHA LEO (Wallace)	Vit. D	Cap.
ROCALTROL (Piramal HC)	Vit. D	Cap.

Vitamin E

BIOE (American Remedies)	Vit. E	Cap.
COVITA (Neo Pharma)	Vit. E	Cap.
ETOPLEX (U.S.V.)	Vit. E	Cap.
EVION (Merck)	Vit. E	Prls./Drp.
EVIT (Abbott)	Vit. E	Cap.
TOCOFER (Torrent)	Vit. E	Cap.
VITEOLIN (Allenburys)	Vit. E	Cap.

Vitamin Combinations of B_1, B_6, B_{12}

ARISTO NEURAL (Aristo)	Vit. B_1, B_6, B_{12}	Inj.
BARAPLEX (A.F.D.)	Vit. B_1, B_6, B_{12}	Inj.
BEDOX (Mesco)	Vit. B_1, B_6, B_{12}	Inj.
BETHADOXIN-12 (Biological E)	Vit. B_1, B_6, B_{12}	Inj./Syr./Tab.
BEVIDOX (Abbott.)	Vit. B_1, B_6, B_{12}	Inj.
MACRABERIN (Allenburys)	Vit. B_1, B_6, B_{12}	Tab.
NEUROBEX (Ind Swift)	Vit. B_1, B_6, B_{12}	Inj.
NEUROBION (Merck)	Vit. B_1, B_6, B_{12}	Inj./Tab.
NEUROKEM (Alkem)	Vit. B_1, B_6, B_{12}	Inj.
NEUROPLUN-12 (Khandelwal)	Vit. B_1, B_6, B_{12}	Inj.
NEUROTON-12 (Mount Mettur)	Vit. B_1, B_6, B_{12}	Inj./Tab.
NEUROTRAT (German Rem.)	Vit. B_1, B_6, B_{12}	Inj./Cap.
NVM (Seagull Labs)	Vit. B_1, B_6, B_{12}	Inj./Tab.
SIONEURON (Albert David)	Vit. B_1, B_6, B_{12}	Inj./Tab.
STAMINE (Stadmed)	Vit. B_1, B_6, B_{12}	Inj.

TRICOMBIN (Uniloids)	Vit. B_1, B_6, B_{12}	Inj.
TRINEUROSOL-H (Merind)	Vit. B_1, B_6, B_{12}	Inj.
VITNEURIN (Glaxo)	Vit. B_1, B_6, B_{12}	Inj.

Vitamin B Complex

BECATONE SYRUP (Alpine)	Vit. B_1, B_2, B_3, Choline, Inositol	Syr.
BECELAC (Pfimex)	Vit. B_1, B_2, B_6, B_9, B_{12}	Cap.
BEPLEX (A.F.D.)	Vit. B_1, B_2, B_3, B_6, Panthenol	Syr./Tab.
BETONIN (Boots)	Vit. B_1, B_2, B_3, B_6, B_9, B_{12}, Calcium Pantothenate	Cap./Syr.
B.G. PROT (Merind)	Vit. B_1, B_2, B_3, B_6, B_{12}	Sol.
COMFORTEX (Recon)	Vit. B_1, B_2, B_3, B_9, C	Cap.
COMPLEX B (Glaxo)	Vit. B_1, B_2, B_3, B_6, Calcium Pantothenate	Tab./Liq.
EBEXID (Sigma)	Vit. B_1, B_2, B_3, B_6, Thyroid Extract	Tab.
ELDERVIT (Elder)	Vit. B_1, B_2, B_3, B_6, B_9	Cap.
HEXAVIT (IDPL)	Vit. A, B_1, B_2, C, D	Tab.
HOVITE DROPS (Raptakos)	Vit. A, B_1, B_2, B_3, B_6, D_3, D, E	Drp.
HYCIBEX SYR (Pharmded)	Vit. B_1, B_2, B_3, B_6, B_{12}	Syr.
MULTIVITAPLEX FORTE (Pfizer)	Vit. A, B_1, B_3, B_9, C, D	Cap.
OPTINEURON (Lupin)	Vit. B_1, B_2, B_3, B_6, B_{12}, Panthenol	Tab./Inj.
PRENATAL (Cyanamid)	Vit. A, B_1, B_2, B_3, B_{12}, C, D, K, Iron, Manganese	Cap.
SURBEXT (Abbott)	Vit. B_1, B_2, B_3, B_6, B_{12}, C, Liver	Tab.
THERAGRAN (Sarabhai)	Vit. A, B_1, B_2, B_3, B_6, B_{12}, C, D, E	Tab.
UNI-VITE (Unichem)	Vit. A, B_1, B_2, B_3, B_6, C, D,	Drp.
VIDALIN (Abbott)	Vit. A, B_1, B_2, B_3, B_6, C, D	Drp.
VI-MAGMA (Cyanamid)	Vit. B_2, B_3, B_6, B_{12}	Drp.
VISYNERAL (USV.)	Vit. B_1, B_2, B_3, B_{12}, C, E	Drp.

Multi-Vitamins

ABDEC (Parke Davis)	Vit. A, B_1, B_2, B_3, B_6, C, D, Sodium Pantothenate	Drp.

BASITON FORTE (Sarabhai)	Vit. B_1, B_2, B_3, B_6, B_9, C	Tab.
BECADEX (Glaxo)	Vit. A, B_1, B_2, B_3, C, D	Tab./Drp./Syr.
BECOSULES (Pfizer)	Vit. B_1, B_2, B_3, B_6, B_9, B_{12}, C, Calcium Pentothenate	Cap./Syr.
BEPLEX (AFD)	Vit. B_1, B_2, B_3, B_6	Inj.
CEBEXIN (IDPL)	Vit. B_1, B_2, B_6, B_{12}, C	Cap./Syr.
DROPOVIT (Wyeth)	Vit. A, B_1, B_2, B_3, B_6, C, D, E, L-lysine	Drp.
EDINOL (Bayer)	Vit. A, B_1, B_2, B_3, B_6, B_9, B_{12}, C, D, E, K, Dried Yeast	Cap.
EMELTONE (Medico Lab)	Vit. B_1, B_2, B_6, Lysine	Syr./Cap.
GUTFLOR (American Rem.)	Vit. B_1, B_2, B_3, B_6, Lactobacillus	Tab.
MYBEX (Medico Labs)	Vit. B_1, B_2, B_3, B_6, Penthenol	Syr.
SANVITONE (Uni Sankyo)	Vit. A, B_1, B_2, B_3, B_6, B_9, B_{12}, C, D, E, Magnesium, Zinc, Fungal Diastase	Cap.
XENEX (Seagull)	Vit. A, B_1, B_2, B_3, B_6, B_{12}, D, Lysine, Zinc	Drp./Syr.

MINERALS

Calcium + Other Minerals

AQUAMIN (Pfimex)	Calcium, Phosphorus, Iron, Magnesium, Zinc, Iodine, Copper, Manganese, Chromium, Selenium, Molybdenum	Tab./Susp.
CALCINOL (Raptakos)	Calcium, Fluoride, Magnesium, Vit. D	Tab.
CAL PLUS (Elder)	Calcium, Vit. D	Tab.
CAL PLUS KID TAB (Elder)	Calcium, Vit. D, Trace Minerals	Tab.
CALCIUM SANDOZ (Sandoz)	Calcium	Inj./Tab.
EFFCAL (Eli Lilly Ranbaxy)	Calcium, Vit. D	Tab.
KALZANA (German Rem.)	Calcium, Vit. C, D	Tab./Syr.
MACALVIT (Sandoz)	Calcium, Vit. D	Syr./Inj.
MATERNA (Emcure)	Calcium, Zinc, Magnesium, Vit. A, B_1, B_2, B_3, B_6, B_9	Tab.

OSIFORT (Systopic)	Calcium, Phosphorus, Zinc	Cap.
OSSIDOSS (Wockhardt)	Calcium, Vit. A, B_3	Tab./Syr.
OSSIVITE (Wyeth)	Vit. A, D, Calcium	Cap.
OSTOCALCIUM (Glaxo)	Calcium, Vit. B_{12}, C, D	Tab.
THERAGRAN M (Sarabhai)	Vit. A, B_1, B_2, B_3, B_6, B_{12}, C, D, E, Iodide, Iron, Copper, Zinc, Manganese	Tab.

Zinc + Other Minerals + Vitamins

BECOZINC (American Rem.)	Zinc, Vit. B_1, B_2, B_3, B_6, B_9, B_{12}, C	Drp./Cap./Syr.
DYNA ZINC (Pfimex)	Zinc	Tab.
STRESS-ZN (Lederle)	Zinc, Vit. B_1, B_2, B_6, B_9, B_{12}, C	Cap.
VIMEZ (Pharmasig)	Zinc, Vit. B_1, B_2, B_3, B_6, B_{12}, Magnesium, Manganese	Syr.
ZENBEX-T (Abbott)	Zinc, Vit. B_1, B_2, B_3, B_6, C, Pantothenate	Tab.
ZIB-C (Mesco)	Zinc, Vit. B_1, B_2, B_6, B_{12}, C	Cap.
ZINFE-SR. (Kal)	Zinc, Iron, Vit. B_6, B_{12}	Cap.

Potassium + Other Minerals

K-GRAD (Wockhardt)	Potassium Chloride	Tab.
POTASOL (Indoco)	Potassium Chloride	Liq.
POTKLOR (Martin & Harris)	Potassium Chloride	Syr.
POTRELEASE (Natco)	Potassium Chloride	Tab./Syr.

Iron Preparations

ANEMIDOX (Merck)	Iron, Vit. B_9, B_{12}, C, D	Cap.
BENOGEN (Rallis)	Iron, Vit. B_6, B_9, B_{12}, C	Cap.
CAPSOVIT (Pharmed)	Iron, Vit. B_9, B_{12}, C	Cap.
CENTOFER-C (Centaur)	Iron	Cap.
CONVIRON (Ranbaxy)	Iron, Vit. B_6, B_9, B_{12}	Cap.
FEFOL (SmithKline Beechem)	Iron, Vit. B_9	Tab.
FEFOL-Z (SmithKline Beechem)	Iron, Zinc, Vit. B_9	Cap.
FERRUM-FOL (Khandelwal)	Iron, Vit. B_9	Tab.
FESOFOR-Z (SmithKline Beechem)	Iron, Zinc	Cap.
FESOVIT (SmithKline Beechem)	Iron, Vit. B_1, B_3, B_6, B_{12}, Sorbitol	Syr./Tab.
HAEM-UP (Cadila)	Copper, Glycerinated Haemoglobin, Zinc	Liq.

HEMFER (Alkem)	Haemoglobin, Iron, Vit. B_9, B_{12}, Zinc, Sorbitol	Liq.
IMFERON (Rallis)	Iron	Inj.
IMFERON B_{12} (Rallis)	Iron, Vit. B_{12}	Inj.
JECTOFER (CFL Pharma)	Iron	Inj.
LIVOGEN (Allenburys)	Liver Concentrate, Vit. B_1, B_3, B_{12}, Yeast	Syr.
MACRAFOLIN-IRON (Glaxo)	Iron, Vit. B_9, B_{12}	Tab.
ROBRAPLEX (Sarabhai)	Iron, Vit. B_1, B_2, B_3, B_6, B_{12}, Pantothal	Syr.
ZEE-NATAL (Pharmed)	Iron, Vit. B_9, B_{12}, C, E, Zinc	Cap.

Oral Electrolytes (Minerals)

ELECTRAL (FDC)	Potassium Chloride, Sodium Chloride, Sodium Citrate, Dextrose	Pdr.
ELECTROBION (Merck)	Sodium Chloride, Potassium Chloride, Sodium Citrate, Dextrose	Sac.
ORALLYTE READY (Mount Mettur)	Sodium Chloride, Sodium Acetate, Potassium Acetate, Calcium Chloride, Magnesium Chloride, Dextrose	Liq.
PEDITRAL (Searle)	Sodium Chloride, Potassium Chloride, Sodium Bicarbonate, Dextrose	Sac.
SPEEDORAL (Roussel)	Sodium Chloride, Potassium Chloride, Sodium Citrate, Glycine, Dextrose	Liq.
WINHYDRAN (Win Medicare)	Sodium Chloride, Sodium Citrate, Potassium Chloride, Dextrose	Pdr.

Minerals + Vitamins

MULTIVITE-FM (Allenburys)	Vit. A, B_1, B_2, B_3, B_6, B_9, B_{12}, C, D, E, Iron, Copper, Manganese, Zinc, Potassium Iodide	Cap.
NUTRISAN (Sandoz)	Vit. A, B_9, B_{12}, C, D, E, Iron, Calcium, Zinc	Cap.

SUPRADYN (Roche)	Vit. A, B_1, B_2, B_3, C, D Tab. E, Calcium, Magnesium, Iron, Manganese, Zinc, Sodium Molybdate, Sodium Borate

AMINO ACIDS

ALAMIN-SE (Albert David)	Essential Amino Acids, Glycine, Sorbitol	Inj.
ALAMIN-N (Albert David)	Essential & Non-Essential Amino Acids, Glycine, Zylitol	Inj.
ALAMIN-SN (Albert David)	Essential and Non-Essential Amino Acids, Glycine, Xylitol	Inj.
AMINO DRIP (Wockhardt)	Arginine, L-Histidine, L-Lysine, L-Tyrosine, L-Phenylalanine, L-Tryptophan, L-Cysteine, L-Methionine, L-Glutamic Acid, L-Hydroxyproline, L-Threonine, L-Leucine, L-Isoleucine, L-Valine, L-Alanine, L-Proline, L-Serine, Glycine, L-Aspartic Acid	Inj.
AMINO PLASMAL-L 5% (Wallace)	Essential and Non-Essential Amino Acids, Sorbitol	Inj.
ASTYMIN-3 (Tablets India)	Essential Amino Acids, Glycine, Sorbitol	Inj.
ASTYMIN FORTE (Tablets India)	L-Leucine, L-Isoleucine, L-Lysine, L-Phenylal-anine, L-Threonine, L-Valine, L-Tryptophan, Methionine, Vit. A, B_1, B_2, B_3, B_6, B_{12}, D	Cap./Liq.
ASTYMIN-C (Tablets India)	L-Threonine, L-Valine, L-Methionine, L-Isoleu-cine, L-Leucine, L-Lysine, L-Phenylalanine, L-Tryptophan	Liq.
HERMIN (Alembic)	Lysine, Threonine, Tryptophan, Leucine, Isoleucine, Phenylalan-ine, Valine, Arginine, Histidine, Glycine, Sorbitol	Inj.
VAMIN-G (Pharmacia)	Mixture of 18 Amino Acids	Liq.

Names of Foods in Indian Languages

English	Hindi	Tamil	Telugu	Kannada	Oriya	Marathi	Bengali	Gujarati	Malayalam
Cereals									
Millet	Bajra	Cambu	Sazzalu	Sajje	Bajra	Bajri	Bajra	Bajri	Kamboo
Barley	Jau	Barli arisi	Barli biyyam	Barli	Jaba dhana	Jau	Job	Jau	Yavam
Buckwheat	Kootu	Kotu	—	—	—	Kuttu	Titaphapur	—	Kootu
Italian millet	Kangni	Thenai	Korralu	Priyangu thene	—	Rala	Syamadhan	Ralkang	Thina
Jowar	Juar	Cholam	Jonnalu	Jola	Janha	Jwari	Juar	Juwar	Cholam
Maize	Makkai; Bhutta	Makka cholam	Mokka jonnalu	Kempu jola	Sukhila maka	Maka	Bhutta	Makai	Cholam
Panivaragu	—	Panivaragu	Varagalu	Baragu	Chinna	Vari	—	Vari	Panivaragu
Ragi (Finger millet)	Mundal	Kizhvaragu	Ragulu	Ragi	Mandia	Nachni	Madua	Ragi	Muthari
Pulses and legumes									
Bengal gram (whole)	Channa	Kothu kadalai	Sanagalu	Kadale	Buta	Harbara	Chola	Channa	Kadala
Split black gram	Urud dal	Ulutham parippu	Minapa pappu	Udina bele	Biri	Uddachi dal	Mash kalair dal	Alad	Uzhunnu parippu
Cow peas	Lobia	Maramani	Bobbarlu	Alasande	Chani	Chavli	Barbati	Chora	Payar

English	Hindi	Tamil	Telugu	Kannada	Oriya	Marathi	Bengali	Gujarati	Malayalam
Field beans	Val	Mochai	Chikkudu	Avare	Baragudi	Walpapdi	Sim	Wal	Val avara
Green gram	Moong	Pasipayar	Pesalu	Hesare kalu	Mooga	Moong	Moog	Moog	Cherypayar
Split kesari	Khesari dal; Lang dal	Kheshari parippu	Lamka pappu	—	Khesari	Lakh dal	Khesari dal	Lang-ni-dal	Vattu parippu
Lentil	Masoor dal	Mysore parippu	Misur pappu	Masur bele	Masura	Masur dal	Masoor	Masur dal	Masur parippu
Moth beans	Moth	Narippayar	—	—	—	Matki	—	Math	—
Peas	Mattar	Pattani	Batani	Batani	Matara	Vatana	Mattar	Suka vatana Pattani	—
Kidney beans	Rajmah	—	—	—	—	Shravan-ghevda	Barbati	Phanasi	—
Split red gram	Arhar dal	Tuvaram parippu	Kanda pappu	Thugare bele	Harada	Tur dal	Arhar dal	Tuver-ni-dal	Tuvara parippu
Soya bean	Bhatmas	—	—	—	—	—	Gari kalai	—	—

Vegetables

English	Hindi	Tamil	Telugu	Kannada	Oriya	Marathi	Bengali	Gujarati	Malayalam
Amaranth, (tender)	Chaulai sag	Thandu keerai	Thota koora	Dantu	—	Math	Notya	Choli-ni bhaji	Cheera
Bathua leaves	Bathua sag	—	—	Sakothina Soppu	Bathua sage	Chandan bathua	Belo sag	Chilni bhaji	—
Betel leaves	Pan-ka pata	Vettilai	Thamala paku	Vilaidyele	Pana	—	Pan	Nagarvelna pan	Vilaidyele

English									
Brussel sprouts	Choki gobhi	Kalakose	—	Mara kosu	Chota bandha gobi	—	Bilati bandha kopi	—	—
Cabbage	Band gobhi	Muttaikose	Gos koora	Kosu	Bhadha kopi Kobi	Kobi	Bandha kopi Kobi	Kobi	Muttagove
Celery	Ajyayan	—	—	—	—	—	Pandhumi sag	—	Sellary
Colocasia leaves	Arvi-ka-sag	Seppam ilai	Chama akulu	Shamagadde yele	Sarue	Alupan	Kochu sag	Alu na patra	Chembu ila
Coriander	Dhania	Kothamalli	Kothimiri	Kothambari soppu	Dhania	Kothimbir	Dhane sag	Kothmir	Kotha-malli
Drumstick leaves	Sajjan patta	Murungai kerai	Muluga akulu	—	Sajnasaga	Shevaga pan	Saj'na sag	Sekta ni sing-no-palo	Murunga ila
Fenugreek leaves	Methi sag	Venthia keera	Menth koora	Menthina soppu	Methi saga	Methi bhaji	Methi sag	Methi bhaji	Uluva ila
Fetid cassia	Chakunda	Togarai	Tantemu	—	—	Takla	Chakunda	Kovariya	—
Garlic	Lassan	Ulipoondu	Velluli	Belluli	Rasuna	Lasoon	Rashun	Lasan	Vellulli
Lettuce	Salad	—	—	—	—	—	Salad pata	Salat	Uvar cheera
Mushroom	Kukurmutta	Kalan	Kukka godugu	—	—	—	—	—	Koon
Spinach	Palak	Pasalai keerai	Bachchali koora	—	Palanga saga	Palak	Palang sag	Palak	Vasala cheera
Tamarind leaves	Imli patte	Puli ilai	Chinta chiguru	Hunise chiguru	—	Chinche-cha-pala	Tetul patta	Amli na patra	Puli ila
Watercress	Chandrasur	Alli ilai	—	Alvi	Brahmi sag	Ahliv	—	Asalai	—

English	Hindi	Tamil	Telugu	Kannada	Oriya	Marathi	Bengali	Gujarati	Malayalam
Beetroot	Chukandar	Beet	Beet	Beet	Bita	Beet	Beet	Beet	Beet
Sweet potato	Shakarkand	Sakkara vali kizhangu	Chilagada dampa	Genasu	Kandamula	Ratala	Ranga alu	Sakkaria	Madura kizhangu
Bitter gourd	Karela	Pavakkai	Kakarakaye	Hagalkai	Kalara	Karle	Karela	Karela	Pavakka
Bottle gourd	Lauki	Suraikai	Anapakaya	Sorekai	Lau	Pandhara bhopla	Lai	Doodhi	Chorakai
Brinjal	Baingan	Kathirikai	Vankaya	Badane	Baigan	Vangi	Begun	Ringena	Vazhuthananga
Capsicum	Simla mirchi	Kodimi lagai	–	–	–	Bhopli mirchie	Lanka (Bilathi)	–	Undamulagu
Cauliflower	Phool gobhi	Kavipoo	Kasu gadda	Hukosu	Phool kobi	Phool kobi	Poolkobi	Phool kobi	Kaliflower
Cluster beans	Guer ki phalli	Kothavarangai	Goruchikudde	Gorikayi	Guanara chhuin	Govar	Jhar sim	Govar	Kothavar
Cucumber	Khira	Kakkarikai	Dosakayi	Southaikayi	Kakudi	Kakadi	Sasha	kakadi	Vellarikka
French beans	Bakla	Beans	Beans	Hurulikay	Bean	Pharasbee	–	Fansi	French avara
Ladies' fingers	Bhindi	Vendakkai	Bendakayi	Bende	Bhendi	Bhendi	Dherash	Bhinda	Vendakka

Onion stalks	Pyaz	Vengaya thandu	Ulli kadalu	Erulli soppu	Piya sandha kakharu	Pati	Piyaz kali	Dunglina dakhadi	Ulithandu
Pumpkin	Kaddu	Parangikkai	Gummadikayi	Kumbola		Lal bhopla	Kumra	Kohlu	Mathan
Sword beans	Bara sem	Kattu thambattam	Adavi thamma	Tumbekai	Maharda	Abaichi sheng	Kathsim	Taravardini vel	Val avara
Round gourd	Tinda	—	—	—		—	—	Todabuch	Thinda

Nuts and Oilseeds

Arecanut	Supari	Pakku	Vakka	Adike	Gua	Supari	Supari	Sopari	Adakka
Cashew nut	Kaju	Mundiri paruppu	Jeedi pappu	Geru beeja	Lanka ambu manji	Kaju	Hijli badam	Kaju	Parangyandi
Coconut	Nariyal	Thenga	Kobbari	Thengini kai	Nadia	Naral	Narkel	Nariyal	Thenga
Gingelly	Til	Ellu	Nuvvulu	Acchellu	Rasi	Til	Til	Tal	Ellu
Groundnut	Moongphalli	Nilakkadala	Verusanagakayi	Kadale kayi	China badam	Bhui moong	China badam	Bhoising	Nilakkadala
Mustard	Rai	Kadugu	Avalu	Sasuve	Sorisa	Mohori	Sorse	Rai	Kadugu
Safflower seeds	Kardi	—	Kusuma ginzalu	—	—	—	—	—	—
Sunflower seeds	Suria muki	Surya kanthi	Poduthiru gaddu puvvu ginzalu	—	—	Surya mukhi	Suraj mukhi	—	Suryakanthi

Fruits

English	Hindi	Tamil	Telugu	Kannada	Oriya	Marathi	Bengali	Gujarati	Malayalam
Bael fruit	Bel	Bilwa pazham	Maredu pandu	-	-	Bel	Bel	Bil	Vilavam pazham
Banyan tree figs	Bargad-ka-phal	Alam pazham	Marripondu	Mara	-	Vada	Bar	Vad	Alam pazham
Cape goose-berry	Rasbari	-	-	-	-	Tipari	Tepari	Popta	Kodine llikai
Dates	Khajur	Pericham pazham	Khajoora pandu	Kharjoora	Khajuri	Khajur	Khejur	Khajur	Eetha pazham
Figs	Anjeer	Atti pazham	Athi pallu	Anjura	Dimiri	Anjeer	Dumoor	Anjeer	Atti pazham
Guava	Amrud	Koyya pazham	Jami pandu	Seebe	Pijuli (deshi)	Peru	Payra (deshi)	Jam phal	Nattu peraka
Jackfruit	Kathal	Pala pazham	Panasa	Halasu	Panasa	Phanas	Kanthal	Phanas	Chakka
Jambu fruit	Jamun	Naga pazham	Neredu pandu	Neralai	Jamukoli	Jambhool	Kalajam	Jambu	Naga pazham
Lemon	Bara nimbu	Pertya elumichai	-	-	Kagaji lembu	Limbu	Pati lebu	Motu limbu	Poonaranga
Lemon, (sweet)	Mitha nimbu	Kolinchi pazham	Gaja nimma parelu	Gaja nimbe	-	-	Mitha lebu	Mitha limbu	-

Lime	Nimbu	Elumichai	Ninma pandu	Nimbe	Gangakulia limbu	Limbu	Lebu	Kadgi limbu	Cheru nuranga
Melon, water	Tarbuj	Darbusini	Puchakayi	Kallangadi	Tarvuja	Kalingad	Tarmuj	Tarbuj	Thannir mathan
Orange	Narangi	Kichili pazham	Kamala pandu	Kithilai	Kamala	Santre	Kamala Lebu	Santra	–
Papaya	Papita	Papalli pazham	Boppayi pandu	Pharangi	Amrut bhanda	Popai	Pepe	Papaya	Omakai
Peaches	Arhoo	–	–	Mara sebu	Piccuu	Peach	Peach phal	Peach	Peaches pazham
Plum	Alubokhara	Alpagoda	Alpagoda	–	–	–	Khajur	–	–
Pomegranate	Anar	Mathalam pazham	Donimma pandu	Dalimbari	Dalimba	Dalimb	Dalim	Dalamb	Mathalam pazham
Custard apple	Sharifa	Seetha azham	Seetha Pphalam	Seetha phalam	Ata	Sitaphal	Ata	Sitaphal	Seetha pazham

Fish, Seafood, Meat and Poultry

–	Bam	Kularal	Mudibo-mmiday	–	Bummi	–	Bam	–	–
Bhetki	–	Painee meen	Pandu chapa	Kolji	Durrah	Khajura	Bhetki	–	Chemballi narimeen
Bombay duck	–	Vangaravasi	Vanamtalu	Bombli	–	Bombil	Nehare	–	Bummili
Catfish	Ashalk machli	Mandai kaleru	Tedijella	Mogam-shede	Shingala	Shingala	–	–	Valla etta

English	Hindi	Tamil	Telugu	Kannada	Oriya	Marathi	Bengali	Gujarati	Malayalam
Folui	Pholi	Chotta valai	Mangali kathi	Pappasi	Pulli	–	Folui	–	–
Kalabasu	Kalabeinse	Kakkameen	Kaki bontha	Kaghi	Kala-beinse	Kanoshi	Kalvus	–	Karthomin
–	Koi	Sennal	–	–	Koi	–	Koi	–	Undeecollee
Magur Pangas	Mangri Pangas	Masaral Kovailoopa-keluthi	Marpoo Choluva jella	–	Magurah Jellum	–	Magur Pangas	–	Yarivahlay
Pomfret, white	–	Mogang vavval	Chanduva	Thondrotte	Bahal	Chandava	Chanda	–	Vella awoli
Singhi	Singhi	Thelimeen thayi-lee	Mapujella	Chelumeenu	Singhi	Bitchuka machi	Singhi	–	Kahree meen
–	Tengra	Auppan keluthi	Yerra jella	–	Kuntiah	–	Tengra	–	Kallan-corree
Rohu	Rohu	–	–	Kanchhi	Rehu	Tambada massa	Ruce	–	–
Sardine	Charee-	Sudai	Kavallu	Pedi; Erebai	–	Pedwa	Khaira	–	Chala mathi
Indian Shard	Hilsa	Ullam	Palasah	Paliya	–	Pala	Hilsa	–	Paluva
Katla	Katla	Theppu meenu	Botchee	–	Barkur	Tambra	Katla	–	Karakatla
Mango fish	–	–	–	–	–	Dodywa; Rawas	Tupsee much	–	–
Prawns	Jinga	Yera	Reyyalu	–	–	Kolbi	Chingri	–	Konch

English									
Sole	Morrul	Virahi	Korra-meenu	Pooli-kuchi	Sola	Sohr	Shol	–	Kannan
Buffalo meat	Bhains-ka-gosht	Erumai iraichi	Barre mamsam	–	–	–	–	–	Pothira-chi
Chicken	Murga	Kozhi	Kodi	–	–	Kombdi	Murgi	–	Kozhi
Goat meat	Khasi ka gosht	Attiraichi	Meka mamsamu	–	–	Bakrya-che mans	Pantar mangso	–	Attiraichi
Liver-(sheep)	Kalija (bher)	Semmari attin eeral	Gorre karjamu	–	Mendha kaliza	Kaleej	Mete (vora)	Kaleju	Semmari attin eeral
Mutton	Bakri ka gosht	Attiraichi	Mamsamu	Mamsa	Manaisa chheli	Mans sheli	Vera mangso	Gheta nu gos	Attiraichi
Pork	Suar ka gosht	Panni iraichi	Pandi mamsamu	Handi mamsa	Ghusuri mansa	Mans (dukar)	Sukar mangso	Suvarnu imas	Panni iraichi

Milk & Milk Products

English									
Milk	Doodh	Pal	Palu	Halu	Dudha	Doodh	Doodh	Doodh	Pal
Curd	Dahi	Thayir	Perugu	Mosaru	Dahi	Dahi	Doyi	Dahi	Thayir
Cottage cheese	Paneer	–	–	–	–	–	Chenna	–	–
Khoa	Khoa	Thirattu pal	Khoa	Khoa	Kua	Khava	Khoa khir	Khoa	Khoa
Butter	Makhan	Vennai	Venna	Benne	–	Loni	Makhan	Venna	Venna
Ghee	Ghee	Ney	Neyyi	Thuppa	–	Thup	Ghee	Ney	Ney

HERBS THAT HEAL
Natural Remedies for
Good Health
H.K. Bakhru

Herbs act in almost magical and astonishing ways — spasms may relax, pains vanish, constipation overcome, nervousness recede, headaches disappear, colds be banished, allergies counteracted, fevers controlled, blood flow arrested . . . the magic is endless.

The book covers more than one hundred herbs, most of which are readily available (some even in your kitchen) or easily obtainable, and describes their specific healing properties, how the herb is useful in alleviating or preventing specific ailments; in most cases, the method of making and using herbal preparations is also explained. Index of ailments which can be treated by herbs makes the book specially useful.

"... a useful hand book."

— The Hindu

"Comprehensive ... recommended."

— Hindustan Times

pp. 240

Rs. 60

HOMOEOPATHIC REMEDIES
FOR MIDDLE & OLD AGE
Dr Keith Souter

For many people either approaching middle age, or in their mid-life, homoeopathy is an ideal method of treatment which accepts reduced physiological functioning of body systems which accompany ageing.

The book covers fifty-seven of the commonest and most beneficial remedies; remedies and treatments that are non-toxic and do not further strain the body systems. It recognises that age-related positive health must necessarily minimise the use of drugs and veer away from the bio-chemical to bio-physical.

Dr Keith Souter, MB, ChB, MRCGP, MHMA, is a practicing GP, homoeopathic physician, part-time University teacher and a medical journalist. He lives in England.

"A well written, well presented and a useful book."

— The Hindu

pp 216

Rs. 110

FITNESS WALKING

Les Snowdon & Maggie Humphreys

Fitness Walking is brisk, rhythmic, aerobic walking — a low impact, low stress form of exercise. When you walk, your BMR (basal or resting, metabolic rate) speeds up and the heart and respiratory rate increases, burning off excess calories, helping you achieve long-term cardiovascular health and fitness.

Fitness Walking helps you regain and maintain your ideal body weight. It improves both muscle tone and strength and you walk away all those flabby areas that you have always wanted to be rid of. It is a totally natural activity which can be enjoyed by all — from the youngest to the oldest. It can be done almost anywhere, at any time and it requires no special skills. It is a fitness for a healthy life.

pp 176   Rs. 125

Available at all bookshops or by V.P.P.

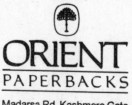

ORIENT
PAPERBACKS

Madarsa Rd, Kashmere Gate
Delhi - 110 006. India